Man Up!

The Ultimate Guide to Natural ED Cures

*Gain Maximum Male Potency
With Guaranteed Solutions Backed by Science
& Powered by Mother Natures Miracles!*

Chad Scott

www.ChadScottCoaching.com

Copyright © 2019 Chad Scott Nellis
All rights reserved. No part of this publication may be reproduced or transmitted in any form or by any means, electronic, or mechanical, including photocopying, recording, or by any information storage and retrieval system.

Table of Contents

INTRODUCTION 1

CHAPTER 1 - AGING IS NOT WHAT YOU THINK IT IS 10

CHAPTER 2 - DO YOU HAVE ERECTILE DYSFUNCTION OR ERECTILE DISSATISFACTION? 16

CHAPTER 3 - SHORT TERM SOLUTIONS DO NOT FIX THE ROOT OF THE PROBLEM 19

CHAPTER 4 - ADDRESS THE ROOTS AND OLD FAITHFUL WILL RISE AGAIN 28

CHAPTER 5 - THE MORE YOU STRESS THE LESS ERECT YOU SHALL BE 37

CHAPTER 6 - SOLID STEEL OCCURS WHEN SECRET AGENTS ARISE.... 50

CHAPTER 7 - THE MAGIC OF TEAM SEX 70

CHAPTER 8 - AS YOU THINK SO SHALL YOU BE 85

CHAPTER 9 - MOTHER NATURE'S MASTER MIRACLES 96

CHAPTER 10 - MOTHER NATURE'S TURBO CHARGERS 112

CHAPTER 11 - THE BIGGEST BONE BREAKER OF ALL 123

THE WORLD NEEDS YOUR HELP! 126

Introduction

Welcome and congratulations on manning up! If you're at all feeling guilty for reading this or wondering if there's something wrong with you, forget it! You, my friend, are not broken!

No, you simply have challenges like every other man. In fact, when it comes to erectile challenges, every man must cross this bridge at some point in their life and there's no shortage of studies to back this up. For example, results from the highly reputable National Health and Social Life Survey (NHSLS) showed the prevalence of sexual dysfunctions (non-specific ED) was 31% among men in the US.[1]

But this survey only scratches the surface. According to a worldwide study researchers estimated that in the year 1995 roughly 152 million men suffered from ED challenges and predicted the number to more than double to 322 million by the year 2025.[2]

And in the UK, according to a study from Atomik research who polled 2,000 men for Co-op Pharmacy, nearly half (43%) of men aged 18-60 across the UK are suffering from impotence.

Sadly, this isn't just affecting guys over 40. In the same UK poll, researchers found 50% of men in their 30's struggled to get an erection compared to 42% in their 40s, 41% in their 50s, and 35% under 30. While these statistics may sound alarming, their ramifications for relationship stability are even more troubling.

Of the respondents, 31% have felt a strain on their relationship as a result of their problems, 31% broke up with a partner due to the issue, 25% lost confidence when dating and 21% suffered mental health problems as a result.

As of now, all statistics point to an epidemic, a sort of plague, which continues to grow out of control without the support of mainstream society.

But There Is Good News!

If any of this sounds familiar, don't worry! Instead, you can take comfort in the fact that in one way or another, at some point in life, every man (and woman) share your dilemma, including top athletes, sages, billionaires, rock stars, presidents and people just like you and me.

Sadly, while every man may experience some form of erection challenge in their life, most do not seek help until its often too late. Instead, they choose to remain on the sidelines sitting on the bench instead of finding a solution and jumping back in the sack.

Multiple studies confirm this as well, including US research, which shows that men with health problems are "more likely than women to have had no recent contact with a doctor regardless of income or ethnicity."[3] Unfortunately, this reluctance means that men often do not seek help until a disease has progressed.[4]

As you might imagine, procrastination can have serious negative consequences. For example, deaths from melanoma are 50% higher in men than women despite a 50% lower incidence of the disease. And while not as life threatening, loss of love in a relationship, as revealed in the UK poll, is more often than not a consequence of not getting help.

So Why Do Men Avoid Seeking Help?

According to another study published by the British Medical Journal, it's not that men don't care about their health; a big part of the problem is that society and health institutions are not set up to cater to men's needs.

For example, women's clinics are quite common while men's clinics are almost non-existent.[5] Social conditioning also plays a role as men are conditioned to believe that being a man means being independent and any attempt to seek help is a sign of weakness.

Nothing Could Be Further From The Truth!

To really "Man Up" means you've made a conscious decision to set aside your fears and become a grower instead of just a shower (no pun intended). Really, the fact that you picked up this book and are seeking answers means you've separated yourself from a majority of men who are either too afraid to seek help or think they're above it (which is really just another way of saying, "I'm scared").

So first off, before we dive in and explore the science and secrets of maximum male potency, it's absolutely critical to get clear about how this book can affect your overall life and give you enough drive to actually implement the tools and strategies recommended. Without this understanding, getting old faithful to rise again will most likely remain an illusion just beyond your grasp.

The Ultimate Goal

This brings us to the ultimate goal of this book and perhaps of life itself, which is to maximize your capacity.

The Ultimate Goal is to Maximize Your Capacity!

So what does maximizing capacity have to do with erections and sex? The short answer is "Everything" but since this goal is absolutely critical to "Manning Up" and getting old faithful to rise again, let's break it down a little further.

Capacity, according to Webster's dictionary is your "ability or power to do, experience, or understand something." Clearly, if you're ability or power to do, experience, or understand male potency isn't currently working, you'll need to step up, grow and increase your capacity.

This not only includes becoming sexually potent but also becoming more courageous, compassionate, wise and intelligent. Essentially, this journey of manning up is about discovering what you're really made of and how you can live up to your full potential.

So get excited because expanding your capacity brings with it treasure trove of rewards and pleasures like better sex, more love, more wealth and robust health.

And if you're at all doubtful that maximizing your capacity is a worthwhile pursuit or life goal, consider the following evidence presented by palliative care nurse Bronnie Ware in her book "Top 5 Regrets of the Dying."

During her many years taking care of the elderly she discovered that the #1 regret of a majority of all men was as follows:

> **"The #1 regret at the end of life is not having the courage to live a life true to oneself but rather, doing what was expected."**

Of course, "true to oneself" is all about making your dreams a reality, which means you won't just be living the status quo and doing what others expected of you. No, to avoid the biggest regret at the end of life you'll need to step up and maximize your capacity and see what you're really made of.

If this sounds intimidating, don't worry! With the right teacher and tools, anyone can make this leap.   And in "Man Up" I'm going to guide you step-by-step to discover some of the greatest rewards and treasures life has to offer with some of the best tools and strategies available.

Who Am I?

I often get queries requesting doctoral credentials for writing a book on a topic like ED, to which I ask, "How many medical doctors have solved your problem with prescriptions and surgery?" Of course, since no medical doctor has ever solved the root problem of ED with surgery or pills they quite quickly shut up.

What's important to understand here is that medical doctors (AKA MD's) don't actually have all of the answers. In fact, the majority of all medical doctors' education and practice is focused primarily on treating the symptoms of a problem rather than the root or underlying cause.   To do this they typically resort to one of two solutions: pills or surgery.

And while surgery can sew your leg back together after an accident or cut out a cancerous tumor, unfortunately, until you address the underlying root of the problem, it's kind of like trying to kill a tree by hacking at the branches. Until you pull out the roots and address the underlying cause, the problem will just keep returning.

Later on we'll talk in detail why short-term solutions work against you, for now, what's important to understand about me is that I'm not interested in how many books you read, podcasts you listen to or doctors you visit. While these can all add value, they don't necessarily treat the root of your problem or create long-term results.

As a certified Master Results Coach with over 12 years of successfully coaching people in life skills and relationships my primary objective is to get new results you can taste touch and feel. Naturally, I do this by addressing the root or underlying cause of the problem, which in turn, creates new results that not only fix your problem for now but for the rest of your life.

I've also been in your shoes and experienced my fair share of erection and relationship challenges. And while our circumstances may differ, I'm quite familiar with the life crushing feeling of overwhelming embarrassment and loss of manhood (perceived, that is).

Fortunately, this challenge pushed me to undergo an extensive study into the root causes of male impotence, the result of which is "Man Up," - an arsenal of incredibly powerful yet simple tools and strategies that have helped thousands of men just like you reignite their sexual potency and zest for life!

My Promise To You

My goal is to support and guide you with the most powerful tools available and help you break through your biggest challenges.

No matter how smart you are, what you look like, what kind of parents you had, where you came from or what your failures of the past may be, if you simply stay open to lifelong learning and take the recommended action in this book, I promise you'll expand your capacity, get new results, find amazing treasures and once again, get your soldier to stand tall and solute her majesty.

Self-Honesty

If fear holds you back and sitting on the couch watching TV seems like a more viable option than expanding your capacity, you may feel comfortable, but you'll most likely never see any of those new treasures, much less learn how to dig them out.

Accordingly, the first step on this journey is to be self-honest about where you're at in life, without which, reclaiming your manhood and sexual power will remain just a dream, like a harem of 10 beautiful women waiting for you in the middle of the Sahara desert.

Tempting as that may seem, its time to wake up my friend, your harem isn't in some far off desert, it's right here in the rewards and treasures you'll find from expanding your capacity. This is your first realization about breaking through and getting your soldier to stand tall once again. So remember this one:

**Self-Honesty Is The First Step In
Getting Your Soldier To Stand Tall**

Because this is so critical to your success, you'll need to make absolutely sure, when you come across certain concepts, tools or strategies in this book, which make you feel a little uncomfortable, instead of retreating to your comfort zone and sitting on the sidelines, be honest about where you're at and know that learning and growing leads to success.

This isn't just hyperbole either. If you read my book "Get High On Confidence" you might remember a study by Dr. Carol Dweck, which found that a growth mindset leads to success, while a fixed mindset leads to stagnation and failure.

Of course, having a growth mindset is directly correlated to maximizing your capacity and if you'd like to learn more about that just head over to my website at www.ChadScottCoaching.com.

It's a Team Effort

Remember I said, "You're not alone?" Not only do guys struggle with sexual dysfunction but women could, in fact, be worse off than men.

Interestingly, in the same study mentioned earlier from NHSLS, researchers found roughly 43% of women reported some type of sexual dysfunction as compared to 31% of men.

So while a woman may never have to worry about boosting a steel pole, she's still human, and as such, will suffer from sexual dysfunction, which means she'll most likely have compassion for your plight and give you a helping hand (more on that helping hand later).

For example, if she has heart disease or is overweight she'll most likely have low libido and her love tunnel will more likely resemble the Sahara Desert than the Niagara Falls.

Yes, women have plenty of sexual dysfunction and will need to look at some of the same root challenges men have if you are to get your team off the bench and onto the playing field. And if your partner doesn't have compassion for your plight, you may want to invest in some couples therapy or reconsider that partnership and find someone else who does.

While this could be interpreted as more bad news, for someone with a "Growth Mindset," this is a great opportunity to solve your problem and create a stronger relationship, so listen very carefully here.

To get your soldier to stand tall, restore your youthful potency and experience an exciting sex life again, it's going to require a team effort. So remember this one:

An Exciting Sex Life Requires A Team Effort!

To do this, you and your partner will both need to commit to making changes, compromising, expanding your capacity and working as a team.

If you're at all opposed to this idea, just know, it's going to be an uphill battle. According to one of the foremost relationship experts in the world, Dr. John Gottman, if expansion and growth are not part of your relationship goals and one or both members of a partnership struggle with self-doubt, you're relationship will be in a constant state of turmoil.

Gottman explains that someone who has "trained his mind to see what is wrong, what is missing and not to appreciate what is there... is what's wrong 85 percent of the time in most marriages."[6]

Essentially, if one person is insecure, with a fixed mindset, they will most likely be judging, disgruntled or dissatisfied with themselves and drive a wedge between you and your ultimate desired goal of a bigger capacity with more love and better sex.

Remember, there is no 'I' in 'Team.' It takes two to tangle and hopefully soon you'll be doing lots of tangling and dangling.

For this reason, I highly recommend you read this book with your partner (or future partner if you're currently single).

Have A Sex Talk

To make any strategy effective and release any unnecessary stress before sex, it's crucial you have a talk with your partner and let them know about the birds and the bees of erection. And hopefully, since you'll be reading this book with them (or buy them their own copy) this is a great opportunity to start the conversation.

You can preface a team-building request with something like:

"Hey I'd really like to ignite our sex life to a whole new level and I found a great book, would you be willing to read it with me?"

Clearly, timing is important when you actually have this talk. You probably don't want to spring this on your partner during breakfast on a weekday when they have loads of responsibilities to think about. Instead, you may want to wait until the weekend or at night when you're relaxing in bed.

If leading with a question sounds a little intimidating, try breaking the ice in a more subtle fashion by picking up this book and reading it in front of her, at which point she'll most likely ask, "What's that all about?"

Since most people are conditioned as children to love and trust those who read them bedtime stories, this could play to your advantage. Naturally, once you start experiment with the strategies in this book there's a really big bonus – a solid pipe and some amazing sex shortly thereafter.

We'll talk more about specific cooperative efforts and how to create the "Winner's Mindset" that leads to more magic in the sack later on. For now, just know you'll need your partner to buy in on this mission.

How To Read This Book

While some of the chapters from this book may not apply to your personal circumstances, each one builds on the next, so on your first pass I encourage you to read all the way through from beginning to end. By reading the whole book you'll be able to identify which challenges may be sabotaging your sexual potency and rule out the ones that are not.

Once you know a particular area could be improved upon, again, make sure you take the suggested action otherwise nothing will change. We'll talk more about the significance of action, for now just know, without it, you'll most likely remain flaccid and continue to experience the embarrassment of rejection and lost manhood.

TIME FOR ACTION!!

To give yourself the best shot at identifying your specific challenge and accompanying solution, commit to finish this book within 30 days or less.

Go ahead and write this goal down in your electronic calendar now. For example: Read "Man Up" every night 8-9 pm for the next two weeks. Don't skip this, go ahead and schedule it now so it's no longer just a dream.

Chapter 1

Aging Is Not What You Think It Is

Most kids look forward to birthdays, often times announcing them to the world so they can celebrate themselves and hopefully in the process get more presents and birthday wishes. But right around the age of 30 to 40 something happens which causes most people to stop looking forward to birthdays and instead dread the thought them.

But Why Do We Lose Our Birthday Mojo?

According to statistics, in the year 2016 the average American watched 270 minutes of TV per day. Of this, we can estimate roughly 20% to be advertisements, which doesn't even account for social media or other publications.[7]

As you can imagine, a large part of our lives are spent being pounded by commercials and advertising, a lot of which conditions us to believe that older is less desirable, less joyful, and can lead to rejection from society.

But the problem is not necessarily the media itself, as media can also function to empower and enlighten. The real problem is the fact that we believe what the media tells us.

And whether you believe the media or not, it's important to understand that cultural conditioning can play a huge role in your beliefs and create horrible results in your sex life. For example, Psychologist Erik Erickson argued that the Western fear of aging keeps us from living full lives and declared:

> "Lacking a culturally viable ideal of old age, our civilization does not really harbor a concept of the whole of life."

Now can you guess what plagues men as one of the greatest contributors to ED?

Fear Is The Mortal Enemy Of Soldier Strength!

Fear, which manifests as stress, creates man down! And while we may have lost any viable ideal of the value of aging and may be missing out on the whole of life, if we simply open our eyes beyond Western Society there is inspiration to be found in many cultures that not only embrace wisdom, knowledge and aging but admire it!

For example, according to the University of Missouri, Kansas City, in Native American families, it's common for younger members to rely upon the elders to pass down their learnings.

Similarly, in Korean society there is great respect and reverence for those with more age and wisdom.

What's even more interesting is the fact that this understanding comes from a belief rooted in the Confucian principle of filial piety. Essentially, filial piety is a fundamental value, which suggest respect for elders and more often than not extends beyond the family and into greater society.

In returning to the importance of cultural conditioning and our beliefs about aging, the great sage and philosopher Confucius himself once declared:

"Few of those who are filial sons and respectful brothers will show disrespect to superiors, and there has never been a man who is respectful to superiors and yet creates disorder."

In other words, order or disorder can in large part be attributed to the respect or disrespect of elders.

While profound and perhaps a subject for an entire book, right now it's important you understand that your age and accompanying wisdom could be the most valuable of all treasures you'll ever acquire in this lifetime.

As far as dreading those birthdays and getting another year older, again, this is just a belief. It's also customary in Korean society to have a big celebration to mark an individual's 60th and 70th birthdays. Perhaps this could inspire more of us to start celebrating our advanced age birthdays? (Yes, naked girls jumping out of birthday cakes are acceptable!)

Regardless of how much you're celebrating or not celebrating, if you choose to believe that getting older is a horrible thing, this belief will cause your soldier to wilt – man down! Fortunately, later on we'll be using some simple, yet powerful techniques to change your beliefs. Right now it's important to open your eyes to the hidden opportunity of getting older and overcoming erectile challenges.

How Can Getting Old And Losing Your Manhood Ever Be A Good Thing?"

Before I answer that question, I'm going to ask you to put aside your inner critic and remind yourself that to fix your problem, you must be open learning and growing by expanding your mental capacity. So go ahead and set aside any potential self-sabotaging thoughts and commit to learning and growing (yep... down there too).

Ready to Expand?

To kick off this magical mystery tour through growth and expansion, we'll start off with your first experience of sexual intercourse.

When recalling your first time having sex you most likely stumbled into that silky tunnel of love and found your pipe throbbing in ecstasy.

Naturally, the first few times you more than likely had no idea how to really put your soldier to work, not to mention, light her up like a Christmas tree, which may have even led to some embarrassment. But once you got that hit of serotonin and oxytocin, no doubt you went back to that velvet tunnel and practiced getting better, maybe even adding in some new techniques, which took your game and partnership to a whole new level of connection and ecstasy.

This first encounter, which was once a challenge, has now transformed into a memorable experience, which in turn has led to growth and new treasures like better sex, self-confidence, less stress and more love.

Since all challenges inherently possess the opportunity to learn, grow and bring out your best, this new phase of re-establishing your sexual prowess is no different.

In other words, experiencing erection challenges is not a death sentence, but rather an opportunity to man up and become a better lover, a more robust, wise and healthy human who is independently confident without the need for approval from others.

This may sound like a lot for someone who just picked up a book looking to find a few penis pick up tricks, but you're about to get way more bang for your buck my friend (pun intended). So celebrate, and make sure you absorb every word like it's your last meal. This desire for growth will catapult you and your big guy to reach the highest of highs (Can you say "erect like Mt. Everest?).

Later on in Chapter 7, we'll talk more about how your beliefs can either propel you to ultimate manpower or sideline your member into drooping depression, for now just know that your challenges are not a problem but an opportunity for growth, expansion and a better sex life.

Personally, I've experienced the hopelessness and depression associated with declining ability to sexually please my woman on several occasions. But instead of allowing it to dictate my life, I educated myself and tested the most effective methods for penile potency both traditional and non-traditional.

After a good 10 years of research and testing, I'm happy to announce the discovery of some groundbreaking solutions that have not only restored a large amount of my youthful potency but also allowed me to increase my capacity to sexually please my woman and give her even greater joy.

The Surprise Attack

While a majority of guys go through their teens, 20s and 30s without a problem getting the big guy to stand tall, eventually something takes us by surprise and completely shakes our foundation; perhaps forcing us to question our manhood.

Confusingly, I found myself no longer able to hold the full erections of my youth, which created a lot of self-doubt and made me feel like I was broken. And worst of all, I didn't have any answers.

It happened right around the time I turned 40 years old when I was dating a 26 year old gal with a large sexual appetite.

I had just come back from a winter surf trip to Mexico tired and drained, but she was revved up and ready to go. When she unexpectedly jumped me, I thought: "Yeah, be a man, crush It!"

Sadly, old faithful wouldn't rise to the occasion like he usually did and I was horribly embarrassed. This episode set off a cascade of negative effects, like more stress, depression and a wedge between me and my gal.

Regrettably, I had just come home from a winter surf trip in Mexico and even though I wore a thick wetsuit and booties, I froze my ass off, I was tired and felt like I was on the verge of getting sick.

Under normal circumstances, getting old faithful to rise wouldn't be much of a challenge. But this time there was no life downstairs. It was as if my license to get an erection had been revoked by some cruel spirit.

No matter what I did (at that point I had no idea what I was doing) I couldn't get an erection and she became very frustrated. Of course, this only made me more self-conscious and crushed the little confidence I had left leaving me unable to perform or communicate. I was mortified, awash with shame, broke down in tears and felt like something was truly broken.

Yeah, I'd heard of guys not being able to "get it up" before but I always thought: "I'll never have that problem, that's for old people or guys who don't take care of themselves." Yet, there I was, "Mr. Healthy," unable to get an erection and satisfy my partner. It was my worst nightmare, like boiling quicksand that sucked me down into a pit of fire and I desperately needed it to end.

It's Natural Don't Sweat It

As traumatic as that episode was, once I learned that sexual slowdown is simply a natural part of the aging process I began to let go of the stress that was killing my potency.

While this might not sound like the first step in solving your erection problems, once you realize you are not alone, the emotional burden and shame that often comes with experiencing erection challenges are minimized. Suddenly, you realize that its not just you, not just your problem and if it eventually affects every man on the planet then it's proof that you are not broken.

But here's the kicker: the emotional consequences of gaining this newfound insight can actually lower your stress levels and help your big guy stand tall. As you just learned, this is really important since one of the biggest factors for ED is stress.

Now before we dive in and find out how to mitigate stress and get old faithful to rise again, it's important to understand where you fall on the roadmap to liftoff. This brings us to our second Chapter: "Do you have erectile dysfunction or erectile dissatisfaction?

Chapter 2

Do You Have Erectile Dysfunction or Erectile Dissatisfaction?

Ok so we now know that no matter what you do and no matter what state of health you're in, all men experience a decline in erectile power and sexual potency as they age. But depending on your lifestyle, your starting point on our journey towards restoring sexual potency will differ from others. For example, someone who is not taking prescription drugs, who is not overweight, will have a very different approach than someone who is overweight and taking prescription drugs.

Unfortunately, both the medical establishment and the general public throw around a lot of confusing terms, which can be misleading, to say the least. So let's dispel any mysteries or misguided information and get you on the right path to health and healing.

The first and biggest misnomer is that Erectile Dysfunction (AKA ED) is the same as Erectile Dissatisfaction. This simply isn't true!

According to the American Urological Association, ED is:

"The inability to achieve or maintain an erection sufficient for satisfactory sexual performance."

If this sounds pretty vague, I'm with you! When I read this definition it sounds like all guys who don't instantly get rock hard erections by looking at a beautiful woman and orgasming exactly when they want all have ED. Problem is, unless you're a trophy winning porn star (if there was one), no guy has perfect control, which according to this definition means every guy on the planet has ED.

But this is really just misinformation and lack of education from the medical community. In order to determine if you have ED the real test is to ask yourself the following question:

Can I Get An Erection From Masturbation?

Specifically, if you have ED it means you're a sober man (no alcohol or other erection-impairing drugs) and cannot raise even a semi-firm erection after extended masturbation. If this is you don't worry, we'll address the most optimal time tested solutions to eliminate ED shortly.   If it's not you the second question to ask is:

What If I Don't Have ED But I Still Have Erection Challenges?

Clearly not every man has ED. According to landmark studies by University of Chicago researchers, among men aged 50 to 64, about one-third suffer from ED and from age 65 to 85, the figure is approximately 44 percent. While ED becomes increasingly common in older men, more than half never develop it.

If you don't have ED but are experiencing erection challenges where your soldier won't stand and salute your gal when she's naked, technically this is called:

"Erection Dissatisfaction"

The fact is, due to the natural process of aging, starting around your late 30's (often earlier among smokers, diabetics and overweight individuals), erections change. In some men, the process is gradual, in others, it happens more quickly. When erections appear, they rise more slowly and do not become as firm as they were during your twenties and thirties; and minor distractions like the doorbell or an ambulance siren may cause wilting.

Sadly, these changes alarm many men, who jump to the conclusion that they must have ED. Fortunately, as just mentioned, if you can still get your soldier to stand tall during masturbation, you don't have ED; what you have is erection dissatisfaction.

Unfortunately, other factors exacerbate erection dissatisfaction, like too much food, anxiety, alcohol, other drugs, relationship problems, and making love when fatigued (remember my winter surf trip).

And while both Erectile Dysfunction and Erectile Dissatisfaction may have similar solutions, they also have some very different ones. So as you read make sure you are absolutely honest about where you lie, otherwise your efforts could be wasted – man down!

What About Impotence?

As for impotence, this term is quite similar to erection dissatisfaction and for most is associated with not being able to sustain an erection. Basically, it's a term for ineffectiveness and like ED gets thrown around haphazardly, creating a lot of fear and misinformation.

What's important to focus on is the distinction between Erectile Dysfunction and Erection Dissatisfaction. Make sure you are clear about which one you suffer from, as this will allow you to accurately choose the solutions that will dig out the toxic roots, reverse your problem and restore your sexual potency.

Now that we got that out of the way I'm going to assume you're now crystal clear on what area your personal challenges lie and it's time to dive into some masterful solutions.

Just keep in mind, not all solutions address the root of your problem and if you fall prey to media hype and commercials that tell you one pill will fix all your problems, I can pretty much guarantee you'll be wasting a lot of time, money and you'll never find any real life treasures. This brings us to our next Chapter "Short term solutions do not fix the root of the problem."

Chapter 3

Short Term Solutions Do Not Fix The Root Of The Problem

Losing the services of your best soldier can be devastating on many levels. Psychological effects, like depression and helplessness, may urge us to make desperate decisions, which can then create negative consequences for our long-term health.

If you think about it, most of life's problems play out in a predictable manner: you have a problem that creates some sort of pain; you want to feel good and avoid the pain so you look for the quickest solution available. You get temporary relief and forget about your pain.

For instance, if you have a headache you may reach for an aspirin, if you're hungry you may look for the quickest snack or if you're on the road, a fast food joint. Or if you suffer from heartbreak you may just look for the first person to love you, etc.

In the case of erectile challenges, you may find yourself searching online or at the doctor's office asking: "What can I do to solve my problem immediately?"

The trap here is the allure of a quick fix, which instead of lightening your emotional load may just lighten your wallet by a couple hundred bucks while at the same time lightening the weight of your stomach as you vomit out those magic pills that somehow made you nauseous instead of instantly erect.

Surprisingly, the problem with this scenario is not the emotional pain of worthlessness, embarrassment, and loss of manhood but the attempt to escape it. As illogical as this may sound, it could be an innovative new solution to your problem; so let me explain.

Ride The Wave Don't Fight It

When I first started surfing over 20 years ago, one of the first things I learned was how to use the wave instead of fight against it. Almost every time I fought against Mother Nature I lost but when I used her power I was able to gain the velocity to stand up and get "barreled" or "shacked" as we like to say in the surf world.

This is the ultimate experience in surfing - when you're in the tunnel of the wave and feel nothing but pure bliss. It's as if time stops as you glide through the cosmos with the rhythm of the universe in the palm of your hands. And... similar to sex, it's quite addictive! (A good addiction at that)

In other words, when you feel the wave of discomfort from embarrassment and rejection or even more trivial waves of boredom and hunger, instead of fighting that pain by trying to numb it or get rid of it with instant gratification from some vice like food, drugs or TV, ride the wave for a bit and take a look at the bigger picture.

Specifically, when you feel the urge for instant pain relief, pause, take a deep breath and ask yourself one of the most important questions you'll ever ask yourself:

What lesson can this experience teach me, which when realized will allow me to harness its power and catapult me forward to greater success?

After asking yourself this question and contemplating it for a bit, more often than not, what you'll realize is that within a short period of time, that urge will pass and give way to a much wider range of choices.

Shortly, we'll talk about that range of choices. For now, just remember, for discomfort from things like hunger and boredom the urge could dissipate within a few minutes but for larger challenges like sexual dysfunction it may be several hours if not days where you'll need to ride the wave.

But this isn't just bro talk for surfers either; this strategy of "Riding the Wave" has actually been proven scientifically to help you find a better long-term solution without the negative consequences of instant gratification.

Research shows that a willingness to think thoughts and feel feelings without having to act on them is an effective method for dealing with a wide variety of challenges such as mood disorders, food cravings, and addiction.[8]

In contrast, if you fight the wave of discomfort by trying to suppress negative thoughts and feelings, like self-criticism, worries, sadness, or cravings, this can lead to even greater feelings of inadequacy, anxiety, depression and even overeating.[9] Ironically, this is exactly the stuff we're trying to avoid.

Armed with this enlightening information, just know from here on out, if you suppress or fight the wave of discomfort by numbing your feelings with instant gratification, you'll only create more pain for yourself. So before you make any desperate moves like buying some magical pills you may later regret, ride the wave for a couple of days before you make a decision.

If you're at all doubtful of my suggestion, perhaps research from scientists at Princeton University will urge you to reconsider.

In a groundbreaking study on predictability, scientists proved that a very small amount of time delaying instant gratification can make a huge difference in helping you make a better decision.[10]

But there's even more good news when it comes to riding waves. Not only does it allow you to learn lessons, expand your capacity and get barreled in her tunnel of love but it also allows you to ditch that whinny little kid in the back of your head that holds you back from manning up!

Even if you don't feel like you have a whinny little kid in the back of your head, chances are, if you're human, you at least have remnants of inner child dysfunction that sabotages your results.

What The Heck Is Inner Child Dysfunction?

Inner child dysfunction represents the failures and traumas of your past, like getting rejected, abandoned, failing in sports or tests, parental abuse, tragic accidents, etc.

What's important to understand is that these events actually hardwire your brain to believe you are unworthy, not good enough, broken or unlovable.

So if you suffer from these disempowered beliefs, when a challenge like erection dysfunction arises, instead of manning up and riding the wave, you may just opt for a blue pill or an injection of some pharmaceutical drug without really considering the consequences.

But this inner child dysfunction could also show up as the whinny little child who never grew up and cries out with thoughts like: give me more, give me more or I don't want to work, I just want to be a selfish blob, sit on the couch and eat Cheetos.

So here's the course correction: when you feel or hear the whiny little kid screaming for instant gratification, if you choose to ride the wave, over time, you'll be able to silence that annoying little kid, man up and get barrelled!

While brain rewiring is a detailed subject I cover in another training called The Winner's Mindset, just know that by repeating this behavior of riding the wave, over time, you will form a new more empowered belief and find yourself looking forward to riding waves.

And more importantly, you'll be able to bypass the pit of self-criticism, worthlessness, and depression and find real solutions that fix your problem long-term. So remember this one:

Whenever you feel compelled to distract yourself with instant gratification, instead take a deep breath, man up and ride the wave!

Not So Magical Pills

Now let's talk about those magical pills for a minute.

If you do find yourself online searching for a quick fix or at the doctor asking for the blue pills, it's absolutely crucial you understand that medical doctors are educated and trained to treat the symptoms of ED and impotence not the underlying causes or root of the problem, which could be a host of other challenges.

Accordingly, I'm going to issue a Warning!

If you take the medical route with pills, creams or devices, just know going in that these are all temporary solutions and without addressing the root, your problem will always return.

That being said, I wanted to make this a fully comprehensive book, which puts all options on the table in order to help you make an educated decision about your personal circumstances.

If you do choose this route, just make sure you're working on the other methods in this book that solve the root of your challenges, otherwise, as you'll soon discover, things could get worse.

The Two Medical Routes For ED

There are two main categories of treatment for ED in the medical establishment - Mechanical and Pharmaceutical. Of these two, pharmaceutical is bar far the most abused and misunderstood. It's also the most prescribed (haphazardly at that) by most medical doctors, so let's unpack this beast and slay it with some truth.

Pharmaceutical Treatments

Confusingly, pharmaceuticals do not address the underlying cause of your problem but instead interfere with the process of blood flow that creates and sustains erections. Essentially, your erect soldier contains up to eight times more blood than when it's flaccid. But once you lose your erection, this trapped blood gets released, your erection ends, and blood flow returns to normal.

PDE5 inhibitors, such as sildenafil (Viagra), tadalafil (Cialis) and vardenafil (Levitra), stop a particular enzyme found in blood vessel walls called PDE5 (phosphodiesterase type 5) from working properly. Since PDE5 helps control blood flow to your pulmonary arteries, PDE5 inhibitors cause your blood vessels to relax, which increases blood flow to your big guy.

Now let's just stop right there. Did you catch that "stop PDE5 from working properly?" Now I don't know about you but I'd rather have Mother Nature working for me than against me (Remember the Wave).

Here's a little food for thought: we do not suffer from erection problems simply because we were not born with enough Viagra in our bodies. Really, can you imagine adding Viagra to the daily recommended allowance of vitamins and minerals needed for survival? Probably not I'd guess. But again, depending on your circumstances, this could be a temporary solution, so let's see what other risks there are before we jump on the Viagra bandwagon.

You're Soldier Could Explode

Turns out these PDE5 inhibitors all have warnings. In fact, here's just one of the many possible side effects copied directly from Viagra's website:

- **An erection that will not go away (priapism).** If you have an erection that lasts more than 4 hours, get medical help right away. If it is not treated right away, priapism can permanently damage your penis.

While you may be saying "whoopee I get a hard on for over four hours," you may want to hold off on that thought. It turns out, holding an erection for long periods of time has actually been proven to do long term damage to your dong. It's called "priapism" and studies show PDE5 inhibitors can "extend duration of action for up to 12 hours."[11]

An extended erection is kind of like staying awake without sleeping for four days and alternating weight lifting with wind sprints - pretty soon your blood vessels will just explode. While that may be a bit of an exaggeration, I think you get the point. Artificially inflated boners for long periods of time are not only detrimental but painful.

They Only Work 50% Of The Time

While manufacturers who sell PDE5 inhibitors promote their drugs as 70% effective, in reality, according to 14 separate studies of over 18,000 men, the success rate is actually closer to 50%. Not exactly an urgent reason to jump off the wave and dive into a bottle of blue pills.[12] And even when these pills do work, don't expect porn-star erections. They only create erections "sufficient for intercourse."

They Create Erections Not Arousal

As effective the PDE5 inhibitors may be for the 50% just mentioned, unfortunately, they have no effect on arousal. So you may get a stiffy, but you may not feel particularly interested in sex. Because of this lack of arousal and other factors, many men feel disappointed with the drugs and according to statistics, fewer than half refill their prescriptions. [13]

They Become Less Effective Over Time

Ever heard of the law of diminishing returns? This happens with all drugs. The more you take them the less effective they become and the more you need to take to get similar effects. Think about smoking pot or drinking alcohol. If you've built up a tolerance, you'll just need more and more to get the same high. Not exactly a good idea considering these drugs have loads of side effects.

There Are Serious Side Effects

And what about those side effects? There are serious negative side effects from taking PDE5 inhibitors that can adversely affect your short and long-term health. Here's a list of some of the manufacturers' warnings:

- Upset stomach or diarrhea
- Dizziness
- Headaches
- Heartburn
- Runny or stuffy nose
- Nosebleeds
- Flushing
- Difficulty sleeping
- Muscle or back pain
- Numbness or tingling in the hands, arms, feet, or legs
- Sensitivity to light or vision changes

Financial Risk

While PDE5 inhibitors have dropped from around $30 a pill to an average price of $7 for a generic brand, it still ads up. And regardless of how much dough you got in the bank, when you consider all the risks, riding that wave to discover some long-term solutions should be sounding pretty stokeworthy about now.

What's The Bottom Line Here?

Given all the risks, pharmaceutical solutions should be a last resort, like when it's your birthday or your partner's birthday and you can't get your pole to rise. Or when you're over 70, in good physical condition, but nothing else seems to work, in which case this may be a good temporary solution.

But even if this is the case, make sure you're addressing the root of the problem; otherwise, you'll just be bailing water from a sinking ship.

Injections

Not so common or painless as popping a pill is the practice of injecting a pharmaceutical substance called alprostadil, which makes your blood vessels expand, allowing for a full, sustainable erection and subsequent panty party. Just keep in mind; this one comes with a big caveat! As you can imagine, injecting anything is traumatic and this one YOU must inject into your own penis. (Ouch!)

Again this is a last resort, a temporary solution. But hey, maybe you're a doctor or you have the stomach for it, in which case you'll mix up a dose, draw it into a syringe then insert the needle directly into a vein in the shaft of your member. Interestingly, with an estimated 80% success rate, this method is slightly more effective than popping a PDE5 inhibitor like Viagra.

Regrettably though, this method may have some undesirable side effects such as painful erections. (Remember priapism?) There is also a suppository version of this medication, which is not often recommended due to its low 30-40% success rate and needless to say - painful application process.

Mechanical Treatments

In some cases, treatment for more severe cases of ED may involve mechanical treatments, such as a penis pump or penile implant surgery.

Penile pumps are devices that are placed over your penis to draw blood into the shaft. Once the vacuum creates an erection through the use of suction, a retaining band is slid down the shaft to the base of your penis to maintain the erection during physical intimacy. This band can be left on for up to 30 minutes at a time.

Pumps can come in two forms, hand operated or battery operated and are also available as prescription or non-prescription models.

Buyer Beware!

If you purchase a non-prescription model, just make sure it has a quick release feature; otherwise, you could be looking at your soldier hanging from the gallows with a long-term injury.

Implant Surgery

Lastly, while some doctors recommend penile implant surgery for extremely severe cases of ED, I don't recommend surgery unless you've had some sort of catastrophic dismemberment of your soldier, in which case you may need to take drastic measures.

If this is not the case, stay focused on the root solutions by address the underlying cause. This, of course, brings us to our next chapter: "Address the roots and old faithful will rise again."

Chapter 4

Address The Roots and
Old Faithful Will Rise Again

We've talked a lot about fixing the root of the problem and now its time to get out your shovel and start digging. Again, if you're just hacking at the branches, taking supplements, popping Viagra or injecting yourself with testosterone, I can pretty much guarantee your problem will continue returning for the rest of your life.

Unfortunately, as you've discovered, there are major drawbacks and unhealthy side effects when you try to solve the effect rather than the root cause of any problem.

To give yourself the best chance at digging out the toxic infected roots that are causing your problem you'll need to "Man Up" and be really self-honest here. Self honesty is always the first step in creating new results, so go ahead and take a deep breath, relax and open your mind as we dig out the root cause of your particular problem.

As we uncover each potential man crusher take a note if any of them resonate with your personal circumstances and try not to skip ahead before you've identified the root cause of your problem. Again, be honest here as it could mean the difference between life and death! As you'll find out shortly, this is not an exaggeration, so listen closely.

Medical Illness or Affliction

Medical causes of ED are among the most common and roughly 90% of cases can be linked in some form or fashion to medical illness or affliction, which is most likely running rampant inside your body.[14]

Some of the more common medical causes we'll be looking at are Heart disease, Diabetes, High blood pressure, Parkinson's disease, substance abuse, prescription medication, injuries to the spinal cord or pelvis and surgical complications.

If you are not in top physical condition or you have not been cleared by a doctor, you may be surprised to find out the cause of your hibernating soldier as one of these challenges, which might not only be causing man down but soon... man dead!

Heart disease

While nobody wants ED, it can serve as an alarm clock - waking you up to the fact that you have heart disease. But don't freak out! This disease can be reversed and we'll get to that shortly. For now, just make sure you're honest about whether or not you experience any of the warning signs associated with this life crusher.

More often than not, heart disease is caused by plaque in your coronary artery or other circulatory systems, which disrupts the flow of blood as it attempts to move throughout your body. This inevitability impairs blood flow to your soldier, making it difficult to maintain an erection.

In fact, this link between heart disease and erectile dysfunction is so common, that often times, when visiting a doctor for ED solutions, he will most likely recommend a heart screening.

This heart screening will determine whether any ED treatment options could potentially exacerbate heart disease and result in a stroke or heart attack. And since heart disease is so often linked to ED it's important to be able to identify the more common symptoms so you can slay this beast before it devours you. Here are some of the most common warning signs:

1) Chest Discomfort
This is the most common sign of heart danger. If you have a blocked artery or are having a heart attack, you may feel pain, tightness, or pressure in your chest. Some people say it feels like an elephant sitting on them and the pain usually lasts for several minutes.

If this ever happens to you, call 911 my friend, you need serious help. If the pain is brief or it's just a spot that hurts more when you push on it, chances are it's not your heart that's the problem.

2) **Pain that Spreads to Your Arm**
Dr. Charles Chambers, director of the Cardiac Catheterization Laboratory at Penn State Hershey Heart and Vascular Institute says, "This pain always starts from the chest and moves outward... but I have had some patients who have mainly arm pain that turned out to be heart attacks."

This is another classic symptom of a heart attack, which radiates pain down the left side of your body. If this happens, again, seek immediate medical attention.

3) **You Feel Dizzy or Lightheaded**
While a lot of things can make you lose your balance or feel faint for a moment, if you suddenly feel unsteady and you also have chest discomfort or shortness of breath, according to Dr. Vincent Bufalino, an American Heart Association spokesman, "It could mean your blood pressure has dropped because your heart isn't able to pump the way it should." Again, if this is you, get help!

4) **You Get Exhausted Easily**
If you suddenly feel fatigued or out of breath after doing something you had no problem doing last week, like climbing the stairs or carrying groceries, this significant and sudden change could be a sign of heart disease – get help.

5) **Snoring**
Snoring while you snooze is not a life threatening disease but unusually loud snoring that sounds like a gasping or choking can be a sign of sleep apnea. This happens when you stop breathing for brief moments at night while you're still sleeping.

Unfortunately, this puts extra stress on your heart and could be a sign of heart disease. If this is you, I highly recommend you get screened for heart disease.

6) **Sweating For No Reason**
Breaking out in a cold sweat for no obvious reason could signal a heart attack. If this happens along with any of the other symptoms just mentioned, call 911 to get to a hospital right away.

If at all possible don't try to drive yourself in any of these situations.

7) A Cough That Won't Quit
While in most cases, this is not a sign of heart trouble, if you have a long-lasting cough that produces white or pink mucus, it could be a sign of heart failure. This happens when your heart can't keep up with your body's demands, causing blood to leak back into your lungs. If this is you get screened.

8) Your Legs, Feet, and Ankles Are Swollen
When your heart can't pump fast enough, blood backs up in your veins and causes bloating or swelling. Heart failure can also make it harder for your kidneys to remove extra water and sodium from your body, which can also lead to bloating.

If you suffer from any of these 8 symptoms just mentioned, make sure you visit a physician to get screened for heart disease and continue focusing on the root solutions, which we'll be addressing shortly.

Diabetes

Diabetes is a disease in which your body is unable to properly use and store glucose (a form of sugar). There are two major types of diabetes, Type 1 and Type 2, both of which can cause ED.

Type 1 Diabetes

Type 1 Diabetes happens when your body completely stops producing insulin. If you're not already familiar, insulin is a key hormone that enables your body to use the glucose found in food for energy. This form of diabetes usually develops in children or young adults but can occur at any age. Sadly, people with Type 1 Diabetes must take daily insulin injections to survive.

Type 2 Diabetes

Type 2 diabetes results when your body doesn't produce enough insulin and/or is unable to use insulin properly (AKA insulin resistance). While this form of diabetes most often occurs in people who are over 40, overweight and have a family history of diabetes, today it's increasingly found in younger people, particularly adolescents.

How Do I Know If I Have Diabetes?

If you have diabetes, chances are you'll experience some of the following symptoms:

- Overwhelming thirst
- Need to urinate more than normal
- Tired and fatigued a lot
- Blurry vision
- Numbness in your hands or feet
- Hungry a lot
- Easily agitated
- Frequent skin, gum or bladder infections
- Wounds that don't heal

In some cases, particularly type 2, there are no symptoms and you could go on for months or even years without knowing you have diabetes. But there is one telltale sign of diabetes and that my friend is... ED!

If your soldier is frequently flaccid and you've been over consuming carbohydrates and sugary drinks for a long period of time, there's a good chance you've done long-term damage to nerves and blood vessels throughout your body. This happens when your body cannot control blood sugar levels (insulin insensitivity).

Sadly, the damage to these nerves and blood vessels prevents your soldier from standing tall even if your hormone levels are balanced and you have the desire to be sexually intimate.

But fear not my friend, by treating the root of your problem with the solutions offer in this book, most of the damage can be reversed. If you're at all doubtful, just keep reading.

High Blood Pressure

High blood pressure, also known as hypertension, means the blood pressure in your arteries is higher than it should be. Often referred to as the "silent killer," hypertension results in a high volume of blood consistently being pumped against your artery walls, which does not circulate properly and can lead to heart problems, kidney failure, and stroke.[15]

Unfortunately, if you have hypertension and your physician prescribes a blood thinning medication like Daimox or Thalidone (boy don't those sound appetizing), your body will not be able to produce the pressure needed to sustain an erection. As a result, you'll experience prolonged episodes of ED for the duration of the time you are on the medication.

Again, you'll need to address the root of high blood pressure in the following Chapters if you are to avoid the pitfalls of pharmaceutical drugs.

Parkinson's disease

Parkinson's disease is a disorder, which affects your central nervous system and the ability to move your body. The symptoms of this disease typically progress slowly, oftentimes with increasing tremors or slowing movement. As time goes on, the symptoms can become more aggressive and begin to affect your facial expressions and speech.

Distressingly, people with Parkinson's disease not only experience symptoms of erectile dysfunction but also decreased libido, premature ejaculation and the inability to orgasm. This is due to the nature of the disease itself as well as a combination of psychological factors that accompany the non-motor symptoms as they begin to progress over time.

Parkinson's and dementia are now increasingly being linked back to the toxification of your body with inflammatory foods, chemicals, and a sedentary lifestyle.[16] So again, handle the root and old faithful will rise again.

Substance Abuse

Substance abuse can have a host of negative effects on your body including Sexual Desire Disorder, Sexual Arousal Disorder, and Orgasm Disorder. Each of these disorders contributes in some shape or form to the larger umbrella disorder of Sexual Dysfunction. Now can you guess what the largest contributor to sexual dysfunction in men is? If you guessed Alcohol abuse, you're right.

Alcohol, Booze, Beer, Wine, etc.

In recalling the poll of 2,000 men from the UK mentioned earlier, we find that 26% attributed their erection challenges to overconsumption of booze. So are they right? Does alcohol really impair sexual potency?

Indeed, it turns out that alcohol is a natural depressant and if you've had too many drinks, chances are your big guy will be demoted to little guy and prevent you from sliding old faithful into the love tunnel.

Unfortunately, men who chronically drink are more likely to experience symptoms of ED due to a consistent depression of their neurotransmitters and their nervous system. This has nothing at all to do with sexual drive, only their ability to act on it.[17]

Accordingly, if you're experiencing symptoms of ED you'll need to take a serious look at your social habits and make sure you are not drinking as a distraction from riding that wave and finding a better solution to a larger issue in your life.

Just know that if this is the case, I got your back my friend. We'll handle this one in Chapter 7.

Smoking

It may come as no surprise, but smoking can also have pervasive negative effects on your manpower. Essentially, when you inhale nicotine it constricts blood vessels and in turn limits the flow of blood to your soldier. So instead of sending him into battle, he'll more than likely get throw into hibernation.

If you're a habitual smoker (cigarettes or marijuana), you've most likely seen the limp dick cigarette cartoons and hopefully had some second thoughts about lighting up. If you're at all doubtful or confused on who to believe, let's shed some scientific sun light on this issue and hopefully raise your soldier back to full salute.

During a clinical animal study aimed at documenting the effects of nicotine on an erection, researchers found the negative effects of nicotine to be so detrimental that they negated the effects of using the PDE5 inhibitor Viagra. Other studies on humans showed that smoking was directly related to low sex drive.[18]

If that isn't bad enough, studies also found 87% to 97% of male smokers have a lower than normal blood supply in their penis.

So if quitting smoking or even moderating it to lower levels is a serious challenge for you, again, keep reading as we'll handle this one in the remaining Chapters.

Surgical Complications

Surgical complications, particularly surgeries performed either directly on or around your soldier (spine or pelvic area), always carry a chance of limiting your ability to get an erection.

While I recommend first approaching this challenge with natural healing modalities, many of these cases will require additional surgery, which will be used to counteract the negative effects of previous surgery.

If this is you, just make sure you've tried the root solutions before you give some doctor the go ahead to begin slicing and dicing you on the operation table.

Prescription Medication

One of life's most vexing paradoxes occurs when we seek out remedies, which may temporarily fix one problem and create another. In the case of ED, many prescription drugs actually create sexual dysfunction.

Many of the most common drugs such as Zoloft and Prozac depress your nervous system and similar to those blood thinning medications for hypertension, wreak havoc, making it difficult if not impossible to produce a functional erection. Even medicine used to help alleviate symptoms for the common cold, such as Sudafed, can have adverse effects on your soldier's ability to report for duty.

If you've been taking a prescription medication for a long time, I highly recommend consulting your doctor or finding a new holistic doctor who can help you wean yourself off of these drugs.

Fortunately, once you discover the underlying root cause of your challenge and begin to slowly remove obstructions to healthy blood flow, your symptoms will reverse and old faithful will rise again.

Most importantly, according to one of the most reputable cardiologists in the world, Dr. Steven Gundry, if you continue to remove obstructions like medications and toxic food, you won't need any prescription drugs ever again. (Can I get a "Hell Yeah!")

Injuries to Pelvic or Spinal Cord

Much like those surgical complications, which can arise from surgery to the pelvic or spinal cord; injuries to these areas can have similar effects.   For example, an injury to your pelvic region can cause vascular damage, which may lower blood flow and deflate your member from actively participating in that panty party.

While an injury may be unavoidable, just know it could indeed be the cause of sexual impotence, in which case you'll need to do all you can to heal up that injury.

This again brings us to our root challenge, which is your bodies' natural ability to heal itself and produce enough blood flow to sustain an erection.

As we dive a little deeper and ride the wave a little longer, we find some not so obvious underlying causes whose roots lie much deeper than just your physical body. This brings us to Chapter 4 "The more you stress the less erect you shall be."

Chapter 5

The More You Stress The Less Erect You Shall Be

Beyond the surface of physical challenges lies a strange and powerful world of wonder where something as simple as a thought can either lift your soldier to full solute or send him into hibernation never to rise again.

Remember the UK poll of 2,000 men from the beginning of this book? Turns out 40% of them blamed stress for their sexual dysfunction.

Stress is indeed one of the most toxic roots that cause ED. But fortunately, we have tools to dig out and eliminate that stress, so pay close attention here, as this could be a game changer for you regardless of your circumstances.

How Do Boners Become Boners?

If you were to look at the underlying process of getting an erection, you would see something like this: Blood rushes in and is sucked up by sponge-like bodies engorging your soldier until he can stand up tall. (Hopefully like the Rock of Gibraltar)

This process happens as a result of sexual arousal when signals are transmitted from your brain to the sensitive nerves in your shaft.

Essentially, being able to get an erection is, in large part, the physical capability of your body's systems to function the way nature intended, i.e. when you're aroused your soldier solutes her majesty.

Sadly, if your mind is not functioning hand in hand with this natural process, your soldier won't solute her majesty and she'll most likely be disappointed.

Personally, I can recall a prolonged period of time struggling with my sex life when I was overrun by financial stress I endured as a struggling musician and entrepreneur. I couldn't pay the rent, I was scraping up change to pay for gas, my dreams were slipping further away and all this stress began to pile up until...

I Got "Dead Dick" (That's DD for short)

Though I didn't fully understand it at the time, the emotional stress I was experiencing was a contributing factor to my inability to man up.

Naturally, after a brief moment of denial, I assumed that my incident was due to aging and lower testosterone. However, as I began to think back to the night of my first occurrence of DD I realized that it wasn't just my physical self, but the mental stress, which had drained me of valuable energy and distracted my thoughts away from arousal and onto problems.

When my girlfriend at the time approached me with the opportunity of a quick roll in the hay, I listened to that small voice in the back of my head saying, "Do what is expected of you" and disregarded the turmoil that was affecting me.

What I did not acknowledge was the fact that I wasn't all in emotionally but instead just went along with what was expected of me. As you can imagine, things didn't turn out so good.

I couldn't get aroused and when my soldier wouldn't report for duty I found both my girlfriend and myself in shock. The resulting disappointment sent me into depression as I wallowed in my failure as a man to please my woman.

Thankfully, I rode the wave and instead of numbing my pain with a bunch of unhealthy distractions I dove into an ocean of research and self-reflection. What I realized was that as we get older, our burdens, whether they be finance, health or relationship issues, become more difficult for our minds and our bodies to bear. We can no longer just push this stuff to the back of our minds and move on like we did when we were younger.

Once you push into your 30's, 40's and beyond the resiliency we once had slows down and new wisdom, tools and strategies are required. Once you grasp this solid dose of reality, there really is nowhere to turn other than to face the truth, man up, expand your capacity and manage your stress.

Worries Wilt Your Wiener

While your story and feelings may differ from mine, all symptoms have a root cause, which when addressed will solve a problem for the long-term. So put your worries aside my friend because these worries could be the biggest obstacle to getting your big guy to stand up tall and go to bat for you. Yes, your worries wilt your wiener and force him into hibernation.

The distinct difference here in Chapter four is this: Your worries relate to the psychological or mental component of erectile challenges and along with emotions such as guilt, fear of intimacy, depression and severe anxiety account for around 40% of all erectile challenges.

Roughly 40% of ED Cases Are Due To Stress

One of the more common traps here is that most men who have ruled out medical conditions but suffer from mental blocks tend to feel like the problem is all in their head, like they just need to "get it together" in order to boost a full erection like they did as teenagers. But this line of thinking only makes your feelings about being inadequate worse and can prevent you from seeking other answers to discovering the root cause of your challenge.

Psychological causes of soldier strength are just as valid as medical causes and need to be considered to begin the healing process and fully take back your penile power.

It's also important to understand that there are many manifestations of childhood and adulthood trauma, which could trigger symptoms of psychological impotence.

But let's tone this down a notch because psychological impotence is really just a fancy term the medical community uses to explain a circumstance where erection or penetration fails due to self-sabotaging thoughts or feelings.

Unfortunately, there's a potential double whammy here as psychological triggers, more often than not, work together, which means it's possible to suffer from several triggers at once. Obviously, not such good news when you're trying to revive your soldier from hibernation.

But remember, an erection starts in your brain with something you think, see or feel and if the signals of pleasure are put on hold by dichotomous thinking or self-doubt, a block to the process is created resulting in an inability to achieve or maintain an erection.

The good news here is that you're not stuck with these thoughts. We'll go into this in detail shortly. Just know for now that by understanding what each trigger means to you and creating a new meaning, you can begin to remove the negative effects of self-doubt and achieve a full solute once again.

Guilt

Many men who experience erectile challenges feel an overwhelming sense of guilt about being unable to satisfy their partners. Psychological studies show that guilt is often paired with low self-esteem, not just in men who experience symptoms of ED but also in men who experience long-standing issues with depression.

Unfortunately, when guilt and self-esteem work hand in hand they create a vicious cycle, which only leads you further down the path of depression and helplessness.

For example, you may feel guilty about not being able to please your partner because of low self-esteem (maybe you failed a lot in the past) but this low self-esteem only multiplies when you add guilt to the equation. If this is you, don't worry; we'll handle this self-sabotaging belief shortly.

Fear of intimacy

The fear of intimacy or that you are somehow incapable of satisfying and pleasing your partner can also cause an inability to sustain an erection.

Often times, these feelings are brought on by years of failure in relationships and other areas of life. This could also manifest as that small voice in the back of your head we talked about earlier – the whinny little kid telling you that you aren't worthy because you were rejected in the past.

These feelings of uncertainty create a lot of self-doubt, which brews and builds into a self-sabotaging time bomb. Sadly, this bomb tends to detonate right before you slug it out of the park and get barreled in her tunnel of love.

If you've read my book Get High On Confidence, you'll have discovered that uncertainty is the opposite of confidence, which means you'll more likely be hearing that small voice again saying something like, "you'll never be able to satisfy her," or "you're worthless don't even try." Again, if you suffer from these challenges, don't worry! I got your back; just keep reading.

Depression

Depression is more than just a simple case of the blues. Rather, depression is marked by long-standing feelings that tend to kill motivation and happiness and linger well beyond an upsetting event.

Some of the most common symptoms of depression include feelings of emptiness or hopelessness, angry outbursts or irritability, loss of interest, feelings of worthlessness and difficulty concentrating. These symptoms make it difficult to even contemplate the thought of sex, much less get a boner.

If you feel you suffer from depression, just know, you're not alone. To some degree, everyone suffers from depression to some degree at some point in their life. The key here is in learning new lifestyle habits that mitigate depression including the redirection of your focus onto beliefs that lift you up into the light rather than pull you down into a dark hole. Yep... we'll handle that shortly.

Stress and Severe anxiety

Similar to guilt and feelings of low self-esteem, stress, and anxiety feed each other in a vicious cycle. Prolonged stress causes anxiety and increased anxiety also contributes to increased stress, which all lead to... "Dead Dick."

When you're under stress your body releases adrenaline, which constricts your blood vessels. Unfortunately, as we learned earlier, increasing blood flow is the key to erection strength so this certainly doesn't bode well for getting your soldier to stand tall.

For instance, when your mind is focused on problems surrounding work, relationships or financial worries, it will be difficult to relax and focus on what is happening in the present moment.

And while a stress response may have been critical to our survival back in Paleolithic times when we ran from predators like tigers and bears, today things are quite different.

Instead of tigers and bears chasing us, we have financial challenges, road rage, and relationship disputes. Sadly, these consistent low dosages of stress eventually build up and lead to burn out, depression and DD.

Since this is so important, let's break it down scientifically so you can understand the important events happening in your body when you have a buildup of stress and a breakdown of sexual potency.

Your Cardiovascular System

When stress occurs, your heart rate and blood pressure, along with stress hormones like cortisol begin to escalate. According to doctors at the University of Rochester Medical School, studies suggest that high levels of cortisol from long-term stress can increase blood cholesterol, triglycerides, blood sugar, and blood pressure, which are all common risk factors for heart disease.

Repeated acute stress and persistent chronic stress may also contribute to inflammation in your circulatory system, particularly in your coronary arteries, which is one pathway that is thought to tie stress to a heart attack. Unfortunately, as we learned earlier, heart disease is a primary contributor to ED.

Your Nervous System

Your nervous system also plays a crucial role in how stress affects your body. The reoccurrence of stressful situations like an overbearing boss or significant other barking out orders can lead to poor functioning of body parts like your most trusted soldier.

While there are several divisions of your nervous system, the autonomic nervous system (ANS) is the key factor in erection power, so pay close attention here.

Your ANS plays a direct role in physical response to stress and is divided into two systems. The first is your sympathetic nervous system (SNS); a system that directly controls your body's fight or flight mechanism.

The second is your parasympathetic nervous system (PNS); which is responsible for restoring, relaxing and healing.

When your SNS is activated, your body shifts all of its energy and resources toward fighting off a life threat or fleeing from an enemy. Your adrenal glands release the hormones adrenaline and cortisol, which causes your heart to beat faster, increases respiration rate, dilates blood vessels in your arms and legs, slows down digestive processes and increases glucose levels (sugar energy) in your bloodstream to deal with the emergency.

The response happens quickly to prepare your body to respond to an emergency situation or acute stress. But once the crisis is over, your body ceases the production of those hormones and in most cases returns to its pre-emergency, unstressed state.

Woefully, chronic stress, which triggers your SNS repetitively, can result in a serious drain on your mind and body forcing your soldier into hibernation.

What Can I Do To Get Rid Of Chronic Stress?

Since the problem of stress overstimulates your SNS, we'll need to counteract this with more stimulation of your PNS, which will allow you to rest, relax, repair and rejuvenate your natural chemical balance, which in turn will increase blood flow to your big guy.

While there are literally hundreds if not thousands of tools, strategies, and techniques available for activating your PNS, meditation and breathwork have been clinically proven through multiple studies to be highly effective as a stress management tool.[19]

If you're at all thinking this is an oversimplified approach to solving erection problems, I can tell you with 100% confidence, as a yoga teacher for over 12 years, people who struggle with stress the most are the ones who can't breathe properly.

People Who Struggle With Stress The Most Are The Ones Who Can't Breathe Properly

Meditation / Breath Work

If you're at all doubtful or the thought of meditation conjures up thoughts of fairy dust and feathers, allow me to show you why this is so important.

Meditation is a practice, which allows you to monitor and control the unproductive thoughts that your mind produces through mental mastery and breath control. Essentially, the biggest benefit of breath control is the fact that it stimulates your PNS and makes you more relaxed, calm and confident, which then allows blood to flow more freely into your big guy.

But the beauty of Meditation is that it extends beyond pole power since it can be practiced anywhere. For instance, you can meditate while you're walking, waiting in line at the grocery store, while you are at work and most importantly... when you get stressed out!

If for example, you are experiencing a lot of stress from work or your relationship, you can immediately interrupt any patterns of negative thinking (remember that whinny kid) by simply breathing deeply through your nose using a technique called Ujjayi Breathing.

Simple Breath Meditation with Ujjayi Breathing

What it is: Ujjayi Breathing is one of the quickest ways to activate your parasympathetic nervous system (PNS) by breathing deeply through your nose with your mouth closed.

The key is to inhale and exhale through your nose with a slight constriction at the back of your throat. Similar to a snoring noise, there is a slight resonation created from this constriction. If you're short on references, just imagine Darth Vader from Star Wars and his constricted breathing. Maybe this is why he was always so calm and collected. I'd also imagine he had some fierce pole boosting ability. Joking aside, if the power of breathwork doesn't make sense quite yet, don't worry; it takes some time to master so just be patient.

How it works: Ujjayi breathing stimulates your PNS by pulling oxygen deep into the lower lobes of your lungs where your PNS is highly concentrated.

While a good yoga class like ones from my Fired Up program will give detailed instruction on incorporating Ujjayi Breathing into your life, you can do this anytime you're stressed, anxious, depressed or as part of a daily practice. But that's not all Ujjayi is good for; it also works wonders for sexual stamina and delaying your orgasms. Yes, you heard me correctly...

Ujjayi Breathing Delays Ejaculation!

I discovered this purely out of experimentation when I was getting down with my girlfriend one day. I was almost at that point of no return, when I thought: "Hey why not just use the Ujjayi technique." As I began to breathe really deeply, almost magically, I went from out of control to back in the thrusters position. And as long as I kept breathing this way, I was like the Energizer Bunny - I just kept going and going and going.

Needles to say, I was able to give her exactly what she wanted until she exploded with joy and crowned me as her hero once again.

While that may sound overly exaggerated, it's really not since biologically, it makes perfect sense. When you use the Ujjayi technique you are stimulating your PNS and relaxing your muscles, including the ones associated with erection and ejaculation.

Effectively, it's the opposite of the constriction of blood vessels when you activate your SNS. And this one little strategy made a huge difference in my sexual performance while winning me huge points with my woman. So take this one seriously and practice it to perfection.

To get you started and prepare yourself for your next opportunity let's practice some Ujjayi breathing right now.

TIME FOR ACTION!

Turn your phone on silent and find a place where you won't be bothered. Either sit in a chair or a cross-legged position on a pillow or blanket preferably with your hips above your knees (for good blood circulation), otherwise, you'll get uncomfortable pretty quick.

Step 1- Nasal Breathing with Resonance

First, we're going to create some resonance when you inhale and exhale. To achieve this, when you breathe in think about creating a slight snoring sound by constricting (slightly closing) the back of your throat.

This isn't a full snore, just enough to create a slight resonance. It may help to lift your tongue to the roof of your mouth on your inhale and let it drop on your exhale.

Now when you do exhale try to say the phrase "HA" with your mouth closed. If you can hear a distinct sound or resonance you're doing it right.

Now go ahead and continue breathing in and out through your nose with your mouth closed and direct this breath into your abdomen or lower belly while constricting the back of your throat.

Step 2 - Feel Your Belly Rise

Put your hand on your belly; you should feel it rise upward when you inhale. As you continue to inhale let the oxygen expand your abdomen and fill your lungs completely, then fill up through your chest, then up into your throat.

To exhale, again you're going close your mouth and try to make the "Ha" sound while allowing the oxygen to slowly release through your nose. Once you start to feel the rise and fall of your diaphragm and you hear a slight resonance from constricting the back of your throat, you're on the right path - keep going.

Step 3 - Lengthen Your Breath 5-10 Seconds

Next, it's time to focus on lengthening your breath by extending both your inhale and exhale. This, of course, translates directly to the activation of your PNS and relaxes your muscles even more - allowing for that delayed orgasm.

To do this, first just count the seconds it takes to inhale and exhale. Your inhale will always be a bit shorter than your exhale so try to inhale for a minimum of 5 counts but shoot for increasing this eventually to 10 counts or more. On your exhale try to extend for 6 seconds or more and again shoot to eventually surpass 10 counts.

Step 4 - Visualize the Ocean Tide

Once you have a good long breath, go ahead and drop the counting and focus on the image of the ocean tide. Do this by creating a moving picture in your mind of the ocean tide traveling in on your inhale and traveling out on your exhale.

Step 5 (Optional) - Add A Mantra

As an alternative, you can add in an optional mantra and think about something other than the ocean tide while breathing.

For example, if you're using your breathwork as a daily practice to lower stress or during sex to delay an orgasm, you can use a mantra or anything that gets your mind to relax and release tension and stress. Here are a few options:

- Peaceful and Centered

- Relaxed and At Ease

- Calm and Confident

This isn't a religious exercise, but if a religious concept, mantra or phrase helps you relax feel free to use it.

Be Patient

If your mind wanders, and it most likely will, remember that any new skill, from playing baseball to having sex, requires time and effort; of course, breathwork is no different.

Ever get distracted when you're trying to focus on one thing? Maybe you were attempting a roll in the hay with your special someone, but you're mind was so worried about giving her the goods and not being rejected that old faithful lost faith and went into hibernation.

Or maybe its time to go to sleep but your mind is spinning in 30 different directions like how you got into a fight with a co-worker or family member, or what an idiot you are for making a mistake on the job.

Make Friends With Distractions

Most people tend to fight the distractions with more negative self talk or numb them with more distractions like drugs, TV and porn.

But I'd like to offer you one of the most ingenious strategies ever created for dissolving distractions. This is really important so listen up!

Instead of fighting distractions or pushing them away, create a partnership and make friends with them. While this may sound counter intuitive, these thoughts are valid and until you see them as such they'll just keep returning to haunt you. So if you struggle with distractions while you're trying to focus on one thing try these three steps:

1) First, just acknowledge distractions and stressful thoughts as valid, they may be telling you something valuable

2) Second, ask what lesson can I learn from these thoughts.

3) Third thank them for the lessons and release them like a cloud floating by never to return again.

For example, let's say you messed up on a work project and you can't forgive yourself, which stews in your mind keeping you up into the wee hours of Count Dracula. First, you say, hey you're valid and I acknowledge you. Second you say, hey is there something you can teach me? (Note: There may not be anything to learn) Third, once you've learned the lesson or just listened to that voice say thank you and release it like a cloud floating by never to return.

Let's Recap!

After you've taken action on the four steps above, you should be breathing correctly and once the Ujjayi sound becomes automatic you'll only have one thing to focus on – step 4 the image (ocean tide) of your breath.

Long Term Habits Take 60-90 Days

You will get better at it, but only if you do it consistently for a good 60-90 days. So make sure you schedule this in your calendar. For a more detailed training on breathing and rewiring your brain, check out The Winner's Mindset.

Chapter 6

Solid Steel Occurs When Secret Agents Arise

Now that you've dug out most of the toxic roots of erection dysfunction and understand how important it is to reduce stress, we're going to dive a little deeper into some more mind body agents, which continue to reduce stress, while building more sexual potency.

Secret Agent #1 - Testosterone

Science has proven time and time again that once a man gets to around the age of 30, a dramatic decrease in the production of the hormone testosterone occurs.[20]

If you're not already in the know, testosterone isn't just responsible for giving us full and frequent erections, it's also the key hormone inside of your body which affects bone and muscle mass, fat storage, the rate of red blood cell production and it even contributes to your overall mood.

Basically, right around the time you enter your thirties, your testosterone production starts to slow down and begins a steady decline. By the time we reach our forties, lower production of testosterone can be felt as a lack of energy, lower sex drive, weight gain, mood swings, and depression.

Do Any Of These Symptoms Sound Familiar?

They should, they are the start of a widely known epidemic known as "the midlife crisis." This is the time in our lives where we are actively looking to reclaim whatever we believed we lost along with our youth.

To compensate we may buy new cars, date younger women, go to more parties, and sometimes even try on a whole new image, all in the hopes that it will take away our negative feelings of "getting older."

More often than not, what we don't realize is that in large part what we are really searching for is a way to replace the testosterone our body no longer produces; so remember this one:

Midlife Crisis Is A Sign Of Low Testosterone

But truth be told, this isn't the only reason for mid life crisis. So let me quickly address the other part which interestingly enough leads us right back to that #1 regret in life we mentioned earlier: Not having the courage to live a life true to oneself but rather, doing what was expected.

If, for some reason, you manage to solve your sexual potency challenges but still suffer from insecurity, self-criticism or depression, I highly recommend checking out my book "Get High On Confidence." This best selling book, will allow you to break free of the chains that hold you back from doing what you really love and can be found at www.ChadScottCoaching.com.

In regards to the testosterone drop from aging, this depends on lifestyle habits and genetics. For example, people age at different rates and so too does the drop in testosterone. But regardless of these differences, your age is not the sole factor in whether or not you experience sexual slowdown and low T.

While men depend on testosterone for things like building muscle, growing a beard and creating a deeper voice, research also shows that weight control can be added to that list.

The Testosterone Weight Connection

Associate clinical professor of urology at Harvard Medical School and director and founder of Men's Health Boston, Dr. Abraham Morgentaler confirms this connection by telling us:

"Multiple studies have shown men with low testosterone have a higher percentage of body fat than men with higher testosterone."

Fortunately, there is good news here as the testosterone weight connection can function in your favor and act as one of the most powerful contributors to stronger erections and sexual performance.

In a 2013 review of weight loss and its effects on testosterone, published in the European Journal of Endocrinology, researchers found that weight loss alone -without testosterone therapy- was associated with increases in testosterone levels.

Additionally, a German observational study published in the journal Obesity found that weight loss was an added bonus for men with low testosterone who were taking testosterone replacement therapy. In summary, the men in this study took testosterone supplements for five years and lost an average of 36 pounds and 3.5 inches off their waists.

So testosterone is clearly tied to your weight. In fact, it wouldn't be much of a stretch to say that:

Your weight and your levels of testosterone are inversely related - when one goes up the other one goes down.

Obviously, there is a point where losing too much weight can be detrimental, but with obesity at epidemic proportions I think its safe to say that if you want your soldier to stand tall, you'll need to get your weight under control.

But before you go out and buy a bunch of testosterone replacement therapy, just know this is also a short-term solution and does not address the root of the problem.

The problem is that physiologically, the relationship between low testosterone and weight gain in men can become a vicious cycle.

Chairman of the urology department at Lenox Hill Hospital in New York City Dr. David Samadi explains:

"Body fat contains an enzyme that converts testosterone into estrogens... Having extra estrogens triggers the body to slow its production of testosterone. The less testosterone you make, the more belly fat you accumulate, and so on and... the more fat you carry around, the faster you'll burn through the already low testosterone levels in your body."

In other words, if you're carrying extra pounds, your testosterone levels will be low and instead of becoming a pussy banging hero you'll more likely be relegated to lazy couching potato.

This is straight talk my friend, because I'm here to help you, not sugar coat things and prolong your pain. So if you really want to get your soldier to stand tall again and solute your woman, listen closely.

If your energy and motivation to get off the couch and burn that fat is low, just know it's only going to get worse. As time goes on, you'll continue to gain weight, melt further into that couch and the days of romping around in the sack will most likely become a memory of the past.

To get you back in the sack and make you a love making hero again, at this point it's absolutely crucial to identify when things start to go south and enact some countermeasures before your mind and body are beyond repair.

To do this I'm going to ask you some important questions, which will shed some light on your challenges and reveal a clear path ahead. Be honest and notice which of the following, if any, apply to your particular circumstance.

- Do you fall prey to the tendency of rationalization by telling yourself "I'm only five or ten pounds overweight," which may have already turned into 15 or 30 pounds?

- Do your everyday tasks, such as walking and climbing steps seem to require more effort to complete than in the past?

- Is your breathing heavy?

- Do you need energy drinks and a lot of coffee because you're tired more often?

- Do you feel like you've lost a lot of your desire to be active?

- Do you overeat and feel stuffed, like you need to take a nap after eating or suffer from heartburn?

If you feel any of the above apply to you, chances are you're overeating, carrying extra weight and it's slowly killing you. Yes, I know that may be strong language, but again, I'm not here to sugar coat things. I'm here to help you learn, grow and set yourself free from the prison of disempowered beliefs.

In regards to food "killing you," it's important we reflect on that for a second, because these symptoms are all similar to the ones experienced by people who are actually on their deathbeds.

Really, just because we are offered excess amounts of food doesn't mean we have to eat it all, nor does it mean we have to starve ourselves in order to adhere to what we believe constitutes a healthy body.

The real challenge lies in being self-honest about our day-to-day habits and identifying which ones help build testosterone and which ones aid in our downfall or relegation to the couch.

When it comes to nutrition, what you think may be contributing to your weight gain may not be what you were taught in high school nutrition or from the Today Show.

For example, the old paradigm of whole grains as the most important food group and fat as the least important has now been officially debunked not only by most doctors but also by the government.

It turns out that eating more healthy fats actually helps you lose weight, while eating excessive carbohydrates makes you gain weight. And when it comes to erections, since we need blood flow, when you eat too much of anything you clog up the pipes and blood doesn't flow.

Nutrition and diet are obviously an in-depth topic with lots of solutions and since it's out of the scope of this training I highly recommend reading Dr. Steven Gundry's "The Plant Paradox," which has helped thousands of people lose weight without having to give up tasty foods. Here's a link to that book on Amazon.

For now, I recommend staying away from all wheat products, as one of its ingredients WGA (wheat germ agglutinin) is a lectin (reactive protein) built into the plant to protect itself from predators. While all plants have these lectins, this particular one can do major harm and according to Dr. Steven Gundry, has been found to cause heart disease and weight gain. Later on in Chapter 8 we'll talk about some specific erection boosting foods.

How Much Can I Eat?

In all honesty, I love food and I look forward to all my meals, but I've learned there are limits, which can either make your life a living hell or an energizing adventure.

When I was in college playing football the goal was to eat as much as possible to become as big as possible. And when I got out of college the goal was to eat whenever food presented itself, which almost always made me sick.

As a result, I struggled with leaky gut for a good 10 years until I finally figured out that not only was I eating the wrong foods but I was eating way too much which made me slow and lethargic.

A big part of the problem with food is that most people operate on a scarcity mindset; they believe that food is scarce and they need to eat as much as they can. While this may have been relevant in caveman days when we went without food for a few days today (at least in Developed Nations) this simply isn't the case.

Food is everywhere you look - in vending machines, at work, at fast food joints, in your car, in the movie theatre, and just about everywhere you can think of.

We are not living in a time of food scarcity, we are living in a time of food gluttony! Accordingly, the biggest challenge is not in getting enough, but taming the beast that always wants more.

Remember that little whinny kid in the back of your head always screaming for more? He needs to be silenced!

So How Much Should I Eat?

In regards to proportions, it's important to only eat enough to fill up 80-90% of your maximum capacity. But why is this important?

Don't Flood The Tank

If you think about what happens when you flood the gas tank of your car it's very similar to overeating.

Prior to fuel injection technology, mechanics would advise: "Don't flood the tank" because it makes ignition difficult to impossible.

Your body is very similar. Eating too much is like activating the kill switch, which turns off your ability to not only walk and talk but to get erect. To make sure you don't overeat and kill the ignition switch, here are a couple simple but powerful strategies:

1) Eat more slowly, as if each bite was your last bite of food on earth – make sure you savor every morsel. This is important because it takes time for the signals of the hormone "Leptin" (Leptin tells you that you are full) to reach your brain.

   By eating slowly you give your hormonal communication system a chance to actually do its job in maintaining balance and order. But if you just shove food down like you're competing with a pack of wolves, chances are you'll overeat every time and regret it.

2) When you first hear that "I'm getting full" voice, stop and leave some room for digestion to occur. By staying just a little hungry, your body will operate much more efficiently and the blood to your big guy will flow more freely.

If you're still not convinced eating less and losing weight is important to your overall health and your sexual performance, just know this: Not only does extra weight make you feel bad on the inside and take the magic out of your wand, but it also makes you feel worse about your physical appearance.

I don't know anyone who wants to appear overweight, wear oversized clothes and deal with the constant shame and embarrassment.   This just piles more stress and depression on top of the already existing low energy and low testosterone from carrying extra weight. So remember:

What if I'm Not Overweight?

If you're not overweight and your soldier still won't stand tall, you may experience other side effects of testosterone deficiency. Below is a list of some of the more common Big T blowouts. As you read them notice if any may be a challenge for you.

- Loss of Body Hair
- Loss of Muscle Mass and Strength
- Weak Bones
- Mood Swings
- Depression

- Hot Flashes
- Low Sex Drive
- Erectile Dysfunction (duh)
- Low Semen Volume
- Fatigue

Because of the simple fact that you're reading this book right now, I'd be willing to wager that you, like most men who struggle with erection challenges, are low on the Big T, which is why I've labeled it "Secret Agent #1."

And while lack of testosterone is a widely known contributor to Erection Dysfunction, Erection Dissatisfaction and Impotence, what most people don't know is that there are natural ways to enhance and boost your testosterone.

And for those singing the mid-life blues, fret not my friend because more testosterone can bring back the vigor of your youth and get your soldier standing tall once again.

We now know that secret agent #1 testosterone, is the master blaster for boosting boners and shortly I'll show you how to produce it in large quantities, but we still have one more secret agent that can lift your soldier, turn back the clock and get you back in the sack. So let's investigate a little further.

Secret Agent #2 - Nitric Oxide

As one of the most sought after elements for male potency, nitric oxide is a powerful molecule that increases blood circulation and is produced by just about every type of cell in your body. It acts as a vasodilator, which causes your blood vessels to expand and dilate and in the process increase blood flow throughout your entire body - including your third leg (yes, that's just another cool way of saying "penis").

What's most crucial about nitric oxide is its ability to boosts boners by thinning your blood and decreasing blood viscosity, which in turn decreases platelet aggregation. Of course, as you learned earlier, you need good blood flow to boost an erection, not to mention reduce your risk of a life-threatening blood clot, which means nitric oxide could be you and your significant other's new best friend.

But it gets even better as nitric oxide is also a primary contributor to fat loss. Essentially, it acts as a powerful anabolic stimulus known to help increase your lean body mass, which allows your body to burn fat for fuel much more easily.

In summary, nitric oxide creates more blood flow to the big guy and it helps burn fat, which allows you to produce more testosterone. Now that, my friend, is synergy in motion!

And if you're feeling the pain of getting older, guess what... Nitric oxide helps with that as well.

Slows Down Aging

According to Dr. Joseph Mercola, "Nitric oxide may also assist with counteracting mitochondrial decline because exercise forces your mitochondria to replicate themselves in response to the higher energy requirement demanded by the workout."

"Even though aging is inevitable, the ability exercise has to spur positive mitochondrial changes may help slow some of the effects of biological aging. Because exercise can promote mitochondrial biogenesis in the brain, it has been shown to positively contribute to the reduction or reversal of age-associated decline in cognitive function and assist in repairing brain damage after a stroke."

Ok, so now we now know the two secret agents for boosting erections, which is more testosterone and more nitric oxide, but here's the million dollar question:

**How can I maximize my levels of these two secret agents and gain back both my youthful vigor
and rock hard erections?**

High Intensity Interval Training (HIIT)

Now before you get intimidated by the words "High Intensity," just know, anyone can do this and later I'll show you how even someone like my 75 year old dad can do it with a body that's been weathered by time.

So put your mind at ease and open your eyes wide please, because this is a game changer for not only your erections but also manning up and living a kick ass life with loads of abundance and fortune.

HIIT is creating an unprecedented revolution in the way exercise has been performed over the last 10 years and there's a good reason. HIIT allows you to work out for less time and achieve more results in a shorter period of time than traditional methods like jogging, aerobics and other forms of exercise.

For example, when you perform conventional cardio like jogging for long periods of time, it's been found to deteriorate muscle tissue and decrease testosterone levels. That's obviously not good, but things get even worse for joggers and cardio enthusiasts.

A study in The American Journal of Physiology found that steady-state cardio decreases the ability of muscles to absorb glucose after training.

Perhaps even more impressive is the fact that HIIT burns fat more quickly and efficiently than any other form of exercise. Did you catch that? Since this is so important I'm going to repeat it.

HIIT burns fat more quickly and efficiently than any other form of exercise

For example, a study at Laval University in Quebec, Canada found that HIIT cardio helped trainees lose nine times more fat than those who trained the traditional way (moderate speed for 20-60 minutes).

HIIT is considered to be much more effective than normal cardio because it alternates the activation of your aerobic and anaerobic endurance systems to multiply the benefits. This constant change in intensity level of exercise is the key to unlocking testosterone, increasing nitric oxide production, shedding unwanted poundage and a whole spectrum of other benefits.

Several studies including one from The Journal of Strength and Conditioning found that HIIT can actually increase free testosterone levels. And remember, that's on top of the testosterone you'll unlock when you shed excess poundage shortly after you begin doing high intensity interval training.

But this is just the tip of the iceberg as HIIT also unlocks the second secret agent to boosting your erections - nitric oxide.

Yes, you can get it from diet, but the real boost again comes from that magical combination of aerobic and anaerobic activity! Several studies back this up including a study published in The Journal of Physiology, which found that six weeks of HIIT on a stationary bicycle led to a 36% increase in endothelial nitric oxide synthase (eNOS) while endurance training over the same time period only led to a 14% increase.

Perhaps one of the most remarkable findings of this study is the massive time savings participants got from high intensity interval training vs. endurance training.

In summary, researchers discovered the endurance group had to cycle for 40-60 minutes 5 times per week to get similar results from the high intensity group, which only had to do 4-6 wind sprints 3 times per week.[21]

Clearly, this is all fantastic news for you, your lady and your sexual performance, but we've got one more really massive benefit of HIIT that arguably trumps them all.

Human Growth Hormone - HGH

Human Growth Hormone (AKA HGH) is kind of like the superhero of hormones.

Remember when you were a teenager and had the power to heal a broken bone in half the time as an adult or boost a boner on command?

That growth and healing power is in large part due to high amounts of HGH and it's responsible for a host of amazing life lifters including:

- Increases Testosterone production
- Improves immune function
- Increased exercise performance
- Better kidney function
- Stronger bones
- Younger, tighter skin
- Fat loss
- Higher energy levels and enhanced sexual performance

- Regrowth of heart, liver, spleen, kidneys, and other organs that shrink with age
- Greater heart output and lowered blood pressure
- Improved cholesterol profile
- Hair regrowth

If you're not already hip to this, just know that as you age, your ability to produce the hormone HGH decreases. By the time you're around 40 years old, your HGH levels will be roughly a third of what they were as a teenager.

Fortunately, according to a study published by the International Journal of Sports Medicine in May 1991, heavy resistance training increased human growth hormone (HGH) in men and women by 200-700%.

Another study from Brunel University in 2003 showed how exercise "training above the lactate threshold may amplify the pulsatile release of HGH at rest, increasing 24-hour HGH secretion". In other words, short bouts of intense training can increase HGH after the exercise and for up to 24 hours.

But the period of time performing HIIT is also important as indicated in a study by Loughborough University which compared the effect of a single 6 second and 30 second sprint on a stationary exercise bike and found a 450% increase in HGH after the 30 second sprint over the 6 second sprint.

Now I'm guessing that after all this compelling evidence you're a little more convinced that HIIT could be the key to unlocking loads of the Big T, nuggets of Nitric Oxide and heaps of HGH, but there are a few more really important benefits you should know about especially if you feel like you're struggling with the depressing effects of age.

HIIT Increases Your Stamina

If you're feeling old or tired, like you just can't last that long, HIIT increases stamina by increasing your VO2 max, which is the maximum amount of oxygen your body can handle while exercising. Essentially, if you're huffing and puffing just walking up the stairs, HIIT can make tasks like this a breeze.

HIIT Reduces Insulin Resistance

Several studies show that since HIIT helps you lose weight, it has a corresponding effect of decreased insulin resistance, which will help you avoid Type 2 diabetes.

Is HIIT The Holy Grail of Boner Boosting Power?

If HIIT isn't the holy grail of "Natural" erection boosting power I honestly don't know what is.

Now remember I said you could put your mind at ease if you felt intimidated by the words "High Intensity?"

Since HIIT is so important, but out of the scope of this book, I did a deep dive into the myriad of ways it can be performed and created an entire course called Fired Up, which shows you exactly how to do it with variations for Low, Medium and High impact.

So if you have bad knees a bad back or haven't exercised in a while, which is how my 75 year old father started, you have nothing to worry about.

Basically, anyone at any age or ability level can do my program and get the holy grail of "Natural" erection boosting power. So if you're interested in finding out more about Fired Up just head over to my website or follow this link here:
www.chadscottcoaching.com/fired-up/

Yoga

Earlier we talked about how important it is to reduce stress, but did you know a regular yoga practice can not only reduce your stress and cortisol but also increase your testosterone levels? If you're at all doubtful or feel yoga is just for women, you're in for a big surprise my friend - just keep reading!

The practice of yoga dates back over 5000 years and is one of the oldest forms of exercise and breathwork known to mankind. More importantly, multiple studies have confirmed that yoga is indeed one of the most effective methods for reducing stress and anxiety.[22]

While this is really good news for us guys with loads of stress, further study conducted by Russian scientists in 2001 examined the effects of the Cobra pose on the hormone levels of seven healthy subjects and found some noteworthy discoveries.

In the experiment, researchers drew blood from a group of seven volunteers both before and after they did the Cobra pose. In their report, they determined that cortisol levels dropped in the volunteers by an average of 11% after holding the pose for 2-3 minutes while testosterone levels increased by an average of 16%, with one male subject experiencing a 33% increase and the lone female in the study experienced a whopping 55% increase.

This is obviously significant as increasing testosterone helps increase libido and lowering cortisol lowers your stress levels, both of which are crucial in getting the big guy to stand tall and salute her majesty.

But What If I'm Not Flexible?

Have you ever heard someone, perhaps even yourself say, "I'm not flexible I can't do yoga?" This is like saying: "I'm not hydrated because I can't drink water."

People are not inflexible because they're just born that way. In reality, babies and children are extremely flexible. The only reason people are inflexible is simply because they do not stretch or do yoga.

Complicating the problem further is the fact that the longer you wait, the more inflexible you become and the more inflexible you become the less you can move. Eventually, if you do not stretch, over time, you may find yourself in some real pain that might not be reversible.

For example, my Dad led a very sedentary life for a long time. He, like most of us, spent a lot of time hunched over while driving, sitting on a couch and slouching over a computer. Eventually, without using counter postures like "Cobra," as mentioned above, his spine fused together in a hunched position.

So unless you want to look like the hunchback of Notre Dame, I suggest you open your mind, man up, expand your capacity and give yoga a shot.

Is Yoga Just For Ladies?

Another widespread misconception about yoga is that it's just for ladies. While in the West it's practiced primarily by women, in India (it's birthplace) the primary practitioners of yoga are men. And if we retrace its history, we find that its pioneers like Patanjali and Iyengar were all men.

The only real reason Western men are just starting to catch on to the incredible benefits of yoga is simply because of stigma. Most men fall prey to the illusion that if women do it, it's probably too feminine, therefore, it can't be good for men.

Nothing Could Be Further From The Truth!

I've been teaching yoga for over 12 years and I'm still blown away by how few guys have caught onto the power of yoga. There's a good reason why It's practiced by media moguls like Russell Simons and Richard Branson, athletes like LeBron James and Ray Lewis, musicians like Sting and Adam Levine, actors like Robert Downey Jr. and people just like you and me - it works!

How It Works

Yoga actually means "union" of mind and body or "connection." Essentially, by creating a regular practice, you'll get the added benefit of developing more mind body awareness.

In other words, you'll start to understand and feel when that stress from your job or relationship starts to shorten your breath and create stress, which normally would've led to some form of illness, disease or DD. But once you are mindfully aware of these triggers you can use yoga to stop their poisonous effects.

Most people know yoga as a form of exercise using a set of postures or poses (aka asana) combined with movement, but this is just one component of yoga. We aren't going to go into a full technical description here, as there are literally hundreds of yoga concepts and schools beyond the scope of this book.

For now, just know that once you practice yoga regularly, you'll start to train yourself to avoid the ravaging effects of cortisol and stress, while building testosterone. And not only does this translate into calm and confident in bed, but sleeping better, increasing your lifespan and ultimately... manning up!

Keep in mind, when you first take a class, you may not like the teacher. They may be inexperienced, too feminine or just not right for you. Sadly, without this knowledge, many people quit soon after their first class.

So if you do choose to take classes at a studio, keep this in mind and keep searching and taking classes with different teachers until you find one that resonates with you.

Alternatively, you can get started today by checking out my Fired Up program, which combines the ultimate synergy and power of Yoga, Strength Training and HIIT. Don't delay on this one, I guarantee you'll thank me one day!

Strength Training

As one of the most well known forms of exercise, strength training also boosts the Big T and builds Nitric Oxide while lowering cortisol and can make a huge difference in your sexual potency.

What It Is - Strength training is a type of physical exercise specializing in the use of resistance to induce muscular contraction, which builds strength, anaerobic endurance, and skeletal muscles. Resistance can be achieved through weights, resistance bands or body weight, so if the gym isn't your thing, don't sweat it because I'm also going to show you how to strength train at home with little to no equipment.

Strength training has been studied extensively and its benefits are one of the most well documented of all exercise methods. Benefits aside, if we just consider daily living, life is much easier and feels better when you're stronger. This plays out every day in common scenarios like carrying your groceries, moving the furniture, carrying your luggage or picking up your gal and throwing her on the bed (sometimes they just like it rough!).

But perhaps even more important is the fact that when you strength train, a host of feel good chemicals like testosterone and serotonin kick in and give you more motivation and confidence to not only go big in the bed but in life.

Let's check out five of the most power packed benefits of strength training so you understand how important it is to sexual potency and actually take action to make it happen.

1) When maximum muscle volume is activated, **strength training builds testosterone more than any other exercise**. Clearly

this is awesome since more testosterone equals better and more frequent erections, energy and cardiovascular health.

2) **It helps you look good naked** by burning fat and losing weight. The more muscle mass you have, the higher your resting metabolic rate. So unlike traditional cardio, strength training causes you to continue burning more calories for up to 72 hours after the exercise through a process known as after burn. This, as you know by now, is a really good thing, since that extra fat you're carrying kills your testosterone and your sexual power.

3) **Turns back the clock**. One study showed that strength training in the elderly reversed oxidative stress and returned 179 genes to their youthful level. In other words, it genetically turned back the clock about 10 years.[23]

4) **Builds a strong heart by increasing blood circulation, lowering blood pressure** and improving cholesterol levels. If you don't already know, heart disease is the #1 cause of death for both men and women in the US and as we learned earlier it is also one of the main contributors to ED.

    According to experts, strength training may be of particular benefit for those with heart disease, which was proven in one study when researchers compared the volume of blood being pumped into the heart from running versus leg presses. Leg presses won hands down.

5) Strength training also **prevents diabetes** by controlling blood sugar and managing energy levels so you don't crash and burn.

Undoubtedly, the evidence is overwhelming. Strength Training, HIT and Yoga create the ultimate synergy of power boosting benefits, which not only make you stronger and more attractive but more alive, youthful, balanced, productive and... sexually potent!

This is exactly why I created the Fired Up program, which combines the synergy of Strength Training, HIIT and Yoga. Again, if you're at all curious to see how it can help you safely, effectively and affordably implement these massive benefits into

your life, check it out at my website here:
www.ChadScottCoaching.com

Rest, Repair & The Big T Boost

Hopefully, at this point, if you've weeded out the root causes of dysfunction, addressed stress, overeating and instituted a program like my Fired Up course, you'll be feeling pretty amazing, but being good to your body doesn't just stop at exercise and nutrition. This is where the rest and repair functions of your body come in big.

It may be hard to believe but sleep is not just something your body does to rest; it's actually an essential time when your body can heal and repair itself. And in our case, Secret Agent #1 Testosterone is manufactured in its greatest quantities while you're dreaming about that harem of 10 luscious babes in the Sahara Desert. So remember this one:

Testosterone Is Produced Mostly When You Sleep!

It's no wonder why 36% of guys from the UK poll mentioned earlier blamed their erection challenges on lack of sleep. Studies have shown that the highest levels of testosterone production happen during REM sleep, which is the deep, restorative sleep that occurs mostly late in the nightly sleep cycle.

Unfortunately, sleep disorders, including interrupted sleep and lack of sleep, reduce your amount of REM sleep and frequently lead to low testosterone levels.

Researchers from Mount Sinai Medical Center in New York have found that men with erectile dysfunction were more than twice as likely to have obstructive sleep apnea as those without erectile dysfunction. This study also showed that the more serious a man's erectile dysfunction, the more likely he was to also have obstructive sleep apnea.

And according to another study published by the Journal of American Medical Association in 2015:

> *"Daytime testosterone levels were decreased by 10% to 15% in a sample of young healthy men who underwent one week of sleep restriction at 5 hours per night, which also happens to be a condition experienced by at least 15% of the US working population."*

If you're getting less than 7 hours of sleep per day, there's a really good chance you're low on the Big T.

Unfortunately, low T isn't the only downside for modeling the vampire lifestyle. In fact, those who are sleep deprived have an increased risk of developing high blood pressure, heart disease, kidney disease, diabetes, and even stroke. And as you learned earlier, the presence of these diseases can lead to symptoms of ED and DD while creating a vicious cycle – man down.

Sadly, the Western World rarely makes sleep a priority but instead favors overindulgence in work, play, vices, and other unhealthy choices. Essentially, if you're neglecting sleep, every part of your life will begin to fall apart including your most trusted soldier.

In validating this claim we find a well-known experiment called the "Russian Sleep Experiment," which showed just how fast your mind and body can begin to deteriorate without the presence of sleep. After two weeks, the sleep deprived subjects of the experiment started experiencing hallucinations and reverted to a more primitive mental state where some even began to consume their own flesh. (Yikes!)

As if eating your own flesh wasn't enough of a shocker to get you to sleep more, maybe this next study will spur you into action or in our case less action and more sleep.

According to research, lack of sleep has been linked to changes in two important appetite-regulating hormones leptin and ghrelin. Shahrad Taheri and colleagues from the University of Bristol analyzed data collected on 1,024 volunteers as part of the Wisconsin Sleep Cohort Study.

The researchers reported in the journal Public Library of Science Medicine that people who consistently slept less than five hours a night had 16% less leptin and nearly 15% more ghrelin than those who were well within the average sleeping time of eight hours a night.

We talked briefly about leptin earlier as in food and increased levels of it, which signal starvation and a need for a bigger appetite, while ghrelin is an appetite stimulant.

In regards to the study just mentioned, the less these subjects slept the more hungry they were, the more food they ate and the fatter they became.

Lack of Sleep Leads To Weight Gain

And as you know by now, the fatter you are, the lower the testosterone you will have, which is directly linked to soldier strength.

The takeaway? Make sure you get around eight hours of sleep every night. If this is a challenge for you, consider investing in some sleeping tools like a white noise machine, meditation program, and yep – Yoga! Remember, yoga has been scientifically proven to reduce stress and stress is one of the biggest culprits for lack of sleep.

Speaking of sleep, there is one amazing chemical that knocks us men out by allowing us to release stress in a massive burst of ecstasy. Can you guess what I'm talking about? That's right – Orgasm, which brings us our next chapter, team sex!

Chapter 7

The Magic of Team Sex

Hopefully, at this point, you've dug out any toxic roots that may be lowering your libido and your secret agents are beginning to help you rise back to lovemaking hero. Once you get to this point, its time to jump back in the sack and go through some real life scenarios of what happens when things go wrong so you can avoid the embarrassment and get it right.

This is the team building part of manning up and creates a great opportunity to not only expand your capacity but fortify your relationship.

How so you say?

If for instance, either you or your sex partner suffer from deep insecurities and are focused on what's wrong or what's missing and lack appreciation for each other, there's a really good chance you'll also refuse to share power and work as a team.

For instance, let's say you jump back in the sack and you can't get your soldier to solute. If you suffer from insecurities, you may not be able to communicate your needs to your partner, at which time you may just feel overwhelmed by embarrassment and shut down.

This is where the "shared power" of a relationship comes in big. More often than not, men feel like they need to dominate and monopolize the power in a relationship. For example, when it comes time to spend money or chose what's for dinner they want to have the final word. Similarly, in sex they feel like they are responsible for all the power that builds an erection, sustains it and gives both parties an orgasm.

Unfortunately, if you currently struggle with insecurity and its resultant tendency to dominate and control your relationship, according to Dr. John Gottman who we mentioned earlier, there is an 81% chance your relationship will self-destruct.[24]

In contrast, if you share power with your partner and she takes some responsibility for your erections and the quality of your sex, then you'll have a much better chance at creating a solution and having amazing sex.

And while it may be tempting to simply pop a blue pill, get an erection and get your rocks off (albeit with loads of side negative side effects) that little blue pill will do nothing to solve any potential underlying insecurity challenges in your relationship.

The good news is, whether your relationship challenges stem from lack of sexual potency or deeper underlying issues, by working to become better in the sack as a team, you'll not only have better sex but create a more loving relationship.

This is so important it deserves your full attention. Are you listening closely? Great, now remember this one:

Team Sex Is The Best Sex

In reality, when it comes to sex, your efforts alone will rarely, if ever, match the efforts of a united team. While there are many reasons a team trumps a solo artist, just knowing that someone's got your back allows you to relax and when you relax you perform better. Remember, when it comes to sex, stress is the enemy and relaxation is your best friend.

Anyone who has performed on stage can attest to this as one of the most critical elements for a good performance. If for instance, you're on stage and stressed out or worried about what the audience thinks, your SNS will kick into high gear, you're palms will grow sweaty and your body will stop working on digestion, and pumping blood to your big guy and instead start diverting oxygen and energy into your limbs so you can fight or run from danger.

So unless you'd rather brawl with your babe, relaxing and sharing power is absolutely essential for great sex to occur. And since repetition is the mother of all skill, this is a good time to revisit the importance of teamwork.

While not mandatory, in order to leap over the hurdles of erection challenges much quicker, I highly recommend you and your partner read and implement the action steps of this guide together. This simple act will not only bring back the magic in your wand but the magic in your relationship, which will bond you on a much deeper level.

Interestingly, this team bonding is also affecting chemicals running through your body and your overall emotional state. According to Larry Young, a professor of psychiatry at Emory

University in Atlanta who studies the role of oxytocin in social bonding:

"When you're first becoming intimate, you're releasing lots of dopamine and oxytocin. That's creating that link between the neural systems that are processing your facial cues, your voice and the reward system."

Essentially, by successfully engaging in team sex over the long term, you'll have a much better chance at sharing power and using teamwork to solve other challenges like finances, health and family issues, which will function to ensure the stability, longevity, and enjoyment of your overall relationship. (Who doesn't want more of that?)

Team Sex Scenarios

Now let's see how we can use some team sex strategies in a few real life scenarios. First, go ahead and recreate the scene of your last embarrassing episode when your soldier suddenly deflated or just wouldn't stand tall.

Got it?

If you'll recall from earlier, we learned that an erect soldier contains up to eight times more blood than when it's flaccid. This is why PDE5 inhibitors, such as sildenafil (Viagra) are so popular and abused - they help you increase blood flow. But you don't need PDE5 inhibitors to get your blood pumping.

Assuming you've handled the root of your problems (mental and/or physical) and you got your testosterone and nitric oxide rocking, you can lift up your pipe with some specific physical actions and a little teamwork between you and your partner.

Amusingly, I learned this strategy when I got into a relationship with a confident and grounded woman who liked to play with herself before we had sex. When she invited me to do the same, my first reaction was, "But that's taboo!"

Happily, after she assured me through some elegant strokes of her love tunnel, my resistance completely disappeared (oh yeah, I also drooled a little out of the crack of my mouth). This act was a revelation of massive proportions and from that point on my whole outlook on the old rules of sexual engagement were destroyed.

In all honesty, prior to this girlfriend, I dated a lot of sexually uneducated women who were unsympathetic to the erection challenges experienced by men. These gals were typically entitled, impatient and expected me to get hard immediately with no intervention. But this new gal was teaching me things I never thought possible, which took my sex life to a whole new level.

What I realized was that I didn't have to succumb to the pressure of getting an auto erection like when I was 25 years old. Instead, I created a new sex modus operandi (SMO), which I'll share with you now. Feel free to take notes or try this on your partner right now (if you have one).

Wet, Wild and Aroused

First, you need to warm her up and get her wet, wild and aroused. To do this, you can employ the use of your hands, lips, and tongue. For maximum arousal, key areas, which are highly sensitive, need to be caressed, kissed and licked.

The most obvious first action here is hand contact, which will then lead to kissing and subsequent tongue twirling.

Some of those key arousal spots include her neck, ears, and inner thighs. This progression will quite naturally lead to the more erotic zones like her breasts, backside, and land of the love tunnel.

For the ladies reading this, you'll need to share power here and become a team player. Specifically, your man possesses some of the same highly sensitive erotic zones you have, which need to be caressed, kissed and licked. We'll talk about the main difference -the magic wand- shortly, so just keep reading.

If tongue twirling sounds a little past your time, hey, let's be real! You may have a long-term partner who you've been with for 30 years and twisting tongues (sober at least) may just be a thing of the past. Or you may only have time for a quickie, which means you may want to bypass the tongue twisting part and just go straight for the goods.

Regardless of where you're at, from a team building perspective, you'll need to talk to each other about when you like to have sex, where your erotic zones are and what really turns you on. Be honest here and most importantly; be open to giving up some power and experimenting with new options.

TIME FOR ACTION!

Get excited because this is what you've been waiting for – Team Sex! This is a great opportunity to fortify the team and win your first sexathon by asking each other some really important questions. Go ahead and read one question at a time to your partner then let them ask you the same question. Try not to interrupt and encourage them not to hold back.

> **When do you like to have sex most?**
>
> **Where are your most erotic zones?**
>
> **What kind of foreplay really turns you on?**

Side Note: This is addressed to the whiny kid in the back of your head who wants instant gratification!

While you may want to dive in pole first and start plowing into the depths of her velvet tunnel within five seconds, don't think for a second, women don't appreciate foreplay. Yes, an occasional quickie keeps things interesting but for the most part, she'll want some warm up time.

So again, silence that little voice - man up and give her some good loving! Now let's move on to a couple more really important questions you need to ask your partner like:

> **What positions do you like most?**
>
> **What sequences of positions do you like most?**

Side Note: Speaking of positions and sequences... remember yoga from earlier? If you still haven't expanded your capacity in this area, you may want to reconsider, as a regular practice will open up a whole new variety of sexual possibilities, postures, and sequences you never even imagined. This takes team sex to a whole new level - Man Up!

Team Sex Strategies

Once you've gotten her sufficiently aroused (hopefully dripping wet) I recommend one of the two following approaches, which can be combined if all else fails to erect your soldier.

Option 1) The Magic Jackhammer

In this first option, The Magic Jackhammer, we'll be using the science of erection and the power of construction to boost a boner that will go the distance. Since we know that blood flow is key to ensuring a steel pipe, we simply need a method that creates enough velocity to engorge your member with enough blood sufficient for penetration. Assuming you've handled the roots of ED challenges, I've create a full proof formula for achieving this goal which works as follows:

More Velocity = More Blood Flow = More Stiffness

The Magic of Lubrication

To get sufficient velocity and break through we'll use the power of the jackhammer in construction as an analogy. While perhaps maintaining a reputation as a nuisance, this handy tool generates enough force and frequency to break through seemingly indestructible concrete.

Similarly, in this first option, you'll need to ask your partner to give you head or stroke your soldier aggressively with enough force and frequency to sufficiently increase blood flow. While not mandatory, I highly recommend some form of lubricant in order to avoid injuring your most valuable player (MVP). This could be saliva, but she'll need a lot of it in order to mimic the wetness of her vagina.

This is super important because the more aggressive they are (without hurting you) the more blood flow will engorge your sword to become a full-fledged steel pipe. And in order to gain enough velocity and make this happen, lubrication is absolutely essential.

Obviously, if she's giving you a hummer, the lubrication will be saliva or edible oil (coconut oil works well) but if she's waxing your sword with her hand you'll need to invest around $8 and get some organic lube. Here's an all-natural solution I recommend you get on Amazon: "Lube Life."

Using Music To Create Optimal Motion

The magic of motion doesn't just stop with your partner giving you the dripping wet jackhammer. To get her up to proper velocity and better ensure a steel pipe erection sufficient for penetration we'll employ the use of another trusty tool – music!

While the rate at which she strokes or blows your magic wand may vary and I encourage experimentation, to get to full engorgement of your soldier you'll need to push up in the range of roughly 140BPM or more (that's beats per minute in music terminology).

Although you can imagine this velocity, to make it simple I recommend turning on some music that reflects this tempo. Here are some examples of songs above 140BPM:

- You and I (Deadmau5 Remix) – 140BPM by Medina Valbek

- Do or Die - 145 BPM by Flux Pavilion & Childish Gambino

- Can't Hold Us - 148 BPM by Macklemore, Ryan Lewis & Ray Dalton

- All I Do Is Win - 150 BPM by DJ Khaled, T-Pain, Ludacris, Snoop Dogg & Rick Ross

Hopefully, by now, you're getting excited just thinking about her doing the wet wild jackhammer on your steel pipe to some Deadmau5. But let's slow down for a second here because you're going to need to educate your partner since she most likely doesn't have much if any, experience with this strategy. So remember:

You must speak up and ask for what you want!

For example, you can tell her something like:

**"Be aggressive and really go for it,
the faster you go the more it turns me on."**

Then follow that up with something like:

**"Just think about Wet and Wild, the more wet,
the more wild, so make sure it's really wet."**

Once you've spoken up, its time to break out the lube so make sure it's close by.

TIME FOR ACTION!

Now it's time to practice team building by verbalizing your needs. Understandably, if you're reading this alone you won't be able to ask questions so I recommend rereading the options above and memorizing them or creating your own.

Just remember, when the next opportunity arises, chances are, if you haven't prepared yourself, you'll just fall into old habits, shut down and suffer from the same poor results.

If you are reading this with your partner, each one of you will need to practice by asking a question like:

How about some team sex tonight?

This can obviously be modified with something a little more fun like:

- **Want to play?**
- **Let's get naked!**
- **Want to jump in the sack tonight?**
- **How about a panty raid?**

The sky is the limit so feel free to get creative; the point here is just to initiate team sex.

Next is the arousal stage, which we already talked about, so assuming you're sufficiently aroused, it's time to communicate your needs. You can start this conversation by asking her to slowly warm you up, and then increase the velocity with something like:

"Go For It Babe, Be Aggressive!"

If she doesn't have perfect technique, which most won't, show her exactly how to stroke the shaft and head of your pipe according to what really turns you on.

Remember, this is a team effort, be patient, relax and laugh, it should be fun! Also, make sure there are no expectations; there is no wrong or right, you're simply experimenting to find the best options.

If you end up having sex and can't read further, don't worry you can pick up where you left off later on.

Option 2) The Magic of Mutual Masturbation (MM)

The Magic of Mutual Masturbation was a gem of inspiration created out of my experience with that confident and grounded woman I talked about earlier who liked to play with herself before we had sex. Since this may be unchartered territory for some, you'll need to take a deep breath and let go of any preconceived beliefs about how sex should proceed.

Essentially, this second option is about manning up by taking things into your own hands (pun intended).

This can be done to start with or as an addition to Option 1 if that doesn't work out. This panty party starts after you've aroused each other with some foreplay, at which point you'll need to man up and say something like:

Hey, can you play with yourself for a minute, it really turns me on?

If you have any reservations about this approach, forget it! This is an outdated belief that is disempowering you from having great sex and I'll prove that to you shortly in the next chapter.

For now, just know that once you engage in MM, no matter how weird it may seem to masturbate in front of your partner, just watching them will most likely turn you into a jaw dropping, saliva dripping, horny hillbilly, which will help your soldier report for duty – like magic!

Why Choose Option 2 over Option 1?

While Option 1 "The Magic Jackhammer," may sound appealing, she may not be able to power pump your soldier to full erection, at which time you'll need to use old trusty - your right hand man. Yes, you'll need to start rubbing the magic lamp and since you've most likely done this more times than I can count, you probably don't need much advice on how to do that.

Don't Forget To Breathe

Remember, too much stress not only kills erections but can make you prematurely eject your baby soldiers. So if you're at all timid or doubting yourself, make sure you relax and breathe deep using the Ujjayi technique we talked about earlier.

If you've taken care of the root causes of ED, all you'll need to do at this point is relax and watch her do her thing while you do yours, at which point old faithful should rise again. Just make sure you've addressed the underlying problems (the roots) of your particular challenge before you attempt one of these solutions.

TIME FOR ACTION!

Time to practice more team sex by engaging in some mutual masturbation. Again, if you're reading this alone you'll simply need to practice verbalizing your needs by repeating the questions mentioned earlier until you memorize them and are prepared the next time you jump back in the sack.

If you and your partner are reading this together, it's time to experiment and have some fun. Go ahead and initiate "team sex" then ask a question like:

Hey can you play with yourself for a minute, it really turns me on?

Next, tell each other how it makes you feel to watch your partner play with themselves. Does it turn you on? If so, don't hold back! Say something like:

Wow, that really turns me on something fierce!

Remember, this is all experimentation, no right or wrong! Your goal here is to have fun, laugh, explore and find the best solution for team sex.

Now guys start waxing your sword, either dry or with some lubricant and ladies you go ahead and get that panty party started. Again, if you have sex and can't continue reading this book, don't worry, you can pick it up later. And hopefully, by now, I've trained you to believe this process is really fun and exciting so I'll be seeing you real soon.

Timing Is Everything

If you've ever gone to bed, tried to have sex and couldn't even boost a banana, but then woke up with a full woody, you may have asked, "Where were you when I needed you most," as if your most trusted soldier had an answer.

Oddly, it turns out that the most common and convenient time for sex is most often the worst time to have sex.

When it comes to erection power, we now know that several critical factors must be in play for your big guy to stand tall including nitric oxide, testosterone, and blood flow.

Now can you guess what's flowing through your veins in the morning more than any other time? That's right, lots of testosterone and hopefully, since you're getting a good 7-8 hours of rest, you'll have an abundance of erection power to play with.[25]

But mornings aren't the only time for highly potent soldier strength. Your testosterone levels are elevated roughly every 3-4 hours during the day. So one hour you may find your battery completely out of juice and a few hours later you may be feeling fully charged and frisky.

For instance, you may feel a little frisky charge right after you eat a nutritious meal, especially if you eat testosterone producing foods and do not flood the tank.

Again, you'll need to have a talk and communicate this to your partner. This is absolutely critical, as the more open and spontaneous you can be, the better the sex you can have.

TIME FOR ACTION!

Here's another team building opportunity. Talk with your partner about the realities of testosterone we just mentioned. For example, depending on your circumstances you could say something like, "I notice I get a little aroused right after lunch, maybe we could romp around in the living room next time that happens. What do you think?"

Next, make an agreement that allows you to both be sexually spontaneous when your testosterone levels are elevated and more compassionate when they're not.

Of course, this isn't just about the guys, ladies you may have some timing issues as well. For instance, you may be menstruating. So while you discuss the testosterone timing make sure you agree to work with any female factors as well.

Here's an example of a hypothetical Sunday afternoon.

Let's say you're watching a game, but you're feeling the rock of Gibraltar rise in your pants or perhaps just a little tingling feeling in your erogenous zone. This is the boost of testosterone, which could be cause for a panty raid.

If you've talked about this in advance and agreed to take advantage of these opportunities, you'll actually act on it and not only have amazing star studded sex, but increase your team bond.

So go ahead and take action by making an agreement for spontaneous testosterone induced sex. Here's an example:

When testosterone is on the rise, as long as we are home and female issues are clear, can we agree to a panty raid?

Sustaining A Stiffy And Going The Distance

Timing isn't just important for the time you have sex but the exact moment of insertion into the tunnel of love.

Think about it: have you ever experienced a time when you got erect but you couldn't sustain it long enough to actually dive in that warm, wet and silky hole? Like maybe you missed your window of opportunity? Or maybe you just couldn't get your soldier to do a full salute and her love tunnel shut down for business.

In the case of the latter, as long as you've used Option 1 or 2 from above she should be good and lubed up, which means you won't need a rock hard erection to slide it in. You'll really only need to be about 80-90% of full capacity in order to guide your magic wand past the entry gate.

Again, wet and wild with lubrication will make all the difference here. Just keep in mind, in order to keep the blood going strong and that erection remaining long, you'll need to pick up the velocity and keep it up.

The Roller Coaster of Love (Tension and Release)

While you may fear the loss of your erection and it may be tempting to bang away with no change in velocity, this could lead to a couple of challenging situations.

First, you simply won't be able to sustain this velocity without premature ejection or your army of soldiers. Second, women don't like to be pounded at high velocity for extended periods of time. Eventually, this can desensitize their feeling of pleasure and possibly even lead to pain from too much friction.

To counteract these pitfalls, but still maintain maximum blood flow, make sure you use tension and release.

A great analogy here is a rollercoaster ride, which gradually edges up a steep hill in anticipation of something big. Then, once you get to the top you accelerate full force down the hill and this cycle repeats itself.

Excitingly, this repetition can be further enhanced by going upside down into a 360-degree loop, which in sex terms could equate to flipping your partner into a new position.

Of course, sex is no different and using this analogy of tension and release could really make the difference between a short disappointing eruption and a long sustained loveathon, which once again builds your bond and solidifies your relationship.

This evidence also supports the use of good music with lots of tension and release. So if you're listening to songs with 140BMP velocity as mentioned earlier, you can slow down a bit when the song slows down and ramp it up again when it hits the chorus.

Breathe Deep To Delay Orgasm

We've all been there! You're pounding away and all of a sudden (Oh Sh*t) you just can't hold back any longer and you prejack (that's shorthand for premature ejaculation).

In order to avoid this potentially embarrassing situation, maintain the magic in your wand, and delay your orgasm, it's absolutely critical to slow down and breath deeply through your nose using the Ujjayi technique we talked about earlier.

Additionally, if you're overstimulated and need more delaying power, pull out and squeeze the tip of your dong to constrict some of the blood which will relax your soldier and keep him on duty.

Eliminate Interruptions

When it comes to missing your window, it's also important to know in advance that any interruption like getting up to get a condom or lubricant could kill your chances of a successful romp in the sack. So before you initiate sex, make sure you've handled the music, lights and your condom and lubricant are within arms reach.

If this is your long-term partner, once she's wet and wild and you're stiff like a pipe, it's time to slide in your magic wand. If you need to use a condom to capture any baby soldiers I recommend first gaining entry bareback and pounding away for a couple of minutes first. Why?

Bareback entry will enable you to get in quicker and pound away until your member is fully engorged with blood, at which time you can reach for the condom and put it on.

If this is a new relationship and you need to start with a condom, make sure it's within arms reach so you can put it on while you're still hard.

What happens if I go flaccid with a condom on?

Don't panic, instead just breathe deep, stay calm and use Option 1 or 2 as mentioned previously until you're really ready. Again, if anything goes wrong (and it will) just remember this formula:

More Velocity = More Blood Flow = More Stiffness

Lastly, if things just aren't working out, this is a sign you lack power in the secret agent department and may just need to take a break to regain your strength. If this is the case, honor it, talk to your partner and agree to be compassionate towards one another when these challenges arise.

Most importantly, have fun, laugh, explore and remember there is no right or wrong; you're simply experimenting to find the best solution.

Have fun, laugh, explore and remember... there is no wrong or right!

If you stick with these strategies, I guarantee you and your partner will see positive if not miraculous results. By engaging in team sex over time, you'll form a new habit, which will start to reinforce sharing power as part of your overall relationship building strategy and love will increase on all fronts. And... you won't even need those blue pills.

Just keep in mind, you'll need to communicate your needs and handle the roots of those underlying challenges. And if you feel awkward in mutual masturbation or insecure about team sex or sharing power, I've got even better news as we are about to move onto Chapter 8 - the most important of all.

Chapter 8

As You Think So Shall You Be

As we move a little deeper into the underlying cause of erection dysfunction and erection dissatisfaction we find perhaps the biggest obstacle of all – your mind.

Fortunately, the mind has been pricked, prodded, excavated and studied for thousands of years with some monumental discoveries, the most important of which could be from roughly 3,000 years ago when the historical Buddha declared:

"What We Think We Become."

Naturally, when a powerful statement like this is proven to work over thousands of years we see multiple masters from multiple disciplines and cultures confirm its credibility. For instance, Bruce Lee, one of the greatest martial artists of all time, confirmed this Master Mantra by declaring:

"As You Think So Shall You Become."

And if the Buddha and a Martial Arts Master don't quite tip the scales for you, consider the late great psychologist Dr. Wayne Dyer who declared:

"As You Think So Shall You Be"

In the psychology world, these mantras are employed by thousands of therapists worldwide, most notably, Cognitive Behavior Therapists (CBT). As a widely used psychological treatment, CBT has helped thousands of people build the confidence to overcome depression, anxiety disorders, alcohol and drug use problems, marital problems, eating disorders and severe mental illness. It may come as no surprise then that the creator of CBT himself, Dr. Aaron T Beck famously declared:

"By Correcting Erroneous Beliefs, We Can End The Overreactions"

Remarkably, of the many masters that subscribed to this mantra, not one attributed their success to their physical features; rather, they credited their success to great mental mastery.

This could be the biggest breakthrough you'll ever experience in reclaiming your youthful potency and rising above the challenges of age related decline. Appropriately, it's important we slow down for a bit to fully absorb this lesson.

Running From The Tiger

When you're in the heat of the moment and your soldier just won't stand tall, more often than not, you're first tendency will be to panic, stress out and think that you're broken, which as you know by know kicks your SNS in high gear, accelerates your heart rate and prepares you for fight or flight.

This experience is like having sex while being interrupted by a burglar who breaks into your house and scares the living crap out of you. Before you can even begin to make sense of things, your most trusted soldier has surrendered. (Help - man down!)

As we mentioned earlier, this stress response was great in caveman days when it allowed us to run away from tigers and bandits and it's great for things like high intensity training. Unfortunately, unless you're on a Safari in the Serengeti of Africa, there is no tiger and instead of the fight or flight response saving your life, it kills your erection and you suffer from the cycle of rejection all over again.

The good news here is that all of this is happening in your mind and if you can gain control over your mind, you can also gain control over your body. If you're at all doubtful, you can put your mind at ease because science has proven beyond a shadow of a doubt that your mind and body are inextricably linked - when you do something to one, it affects the other.[26]

Now assuming you've handled all the above challenges and dug out the toxic roots of what is actually blocking blood flow and stealing the magic from your wand, its time to learn how you can get an erection no matter how flaccid your favorite friend is under any circumstance.

The fact is, if you believe and think you're broken or there is something wrong with you, you're mind will communicate this to your body and shut down your soldier quicker than a needle in a balloon.

The Circle of Results Model

Accordingly, to change any disempowering beliefs that pop your balloon and steal your magic were going to use one of the most masterful tools ever created called "The Circle of Results Model."

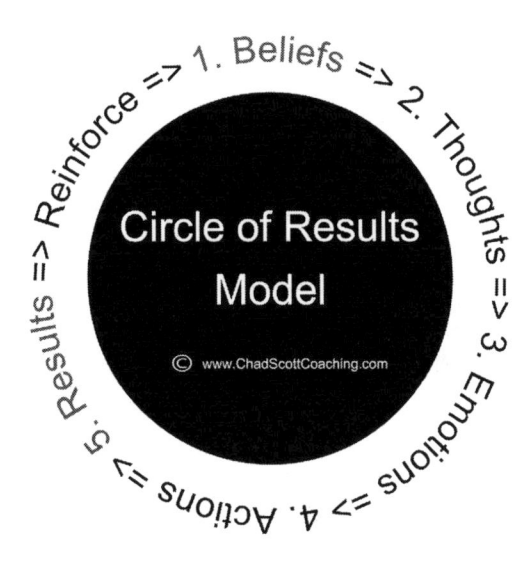

Circle of Results Model
1. Beliefs => 2. Thoughts => 3. Emotions => 4. Actions => 5. Results => Reinforce =>

As you can see from the Circle of Results Model diagram, a belief creates a chain reaction, which ultimately leads to a result as follows:

Beliefs   => Thoughts
Thoughts => Emotions
Emotions => Actions
Actions   => Results
Results   => Reinforce Beliefs

Think about that for a second. Each time you reinforce some behavior like thinking, "I'm a failure" or "I'm broken" or "mutual masturbation is embarrassing" over and over; it actually reinforces your disempowered belief and gets hard-wired into your brain as a negative belief. And the more you do this, the more difficult it is to undo or rewire this belief.

If you've read any of my previous books you most likely remember this statement: "Neurons that fire together wire together," which was also made famous by Dr. Joe Dispenza a neuroscientist in the movie "What the Bleep Do We Know."

This is how your brain works. Your neurons in your brain are the wires that connect associated memories with experiences you've had in the past, which then create your beliefs.

So if you believe every time you get naked with a woman you experience DD (because this did in fact happen several times and embarrassed you) then your brain will fire off the association wires of "sex" equals "embarrassed and broken" and strengthen its bond.

Neurological Repatterning

Unfortunately, by habitually thinking the same negative thing over and over you create what we call a negative thought pattern. To understand how this works we'll use the timeless analogy of a broken record.

Imagine a record is scratched and one phrase plays over and over. This phrase would represent your current disempowered belief or negative thought pattern. Let's say the belief is that you cannot get an erection because you're broken or you're too old.

Each time you are presented with an opportunity to have sex, that broken record kicks in and says, no you aren't capable, don't bother it's not going to get hard! Problem is, this negative pattern reinforces the neural connections in your brain associated with this memory of failure. And the result - the broken record continues to create poor results and make your life miserable (man down).

But if you can create a new groove in the record with a newly empowered belief, you'll get a different result (man up). Below

I've listed a few examples of empowered beliefs, as you read them notice which ones resonate most for you.

- I am calm and confident, I believe if I just take my time I'll give her so much pleasure she'll forget her own name and crown me king.

- I believe my age is an asset, it gives me more patience; I believe when I take it slower it lasts longer and feels better.

- I believe my erection challenges are a natural part of aging and create an opportunity to strengthen my bond with my partner, have better sex and get even more love.

Quite amazingly, by repeating a newly empowered belief, over time, you can interrupt negative thought patterns and change your belief. In the Neuro Linguistic Programming (NLP) world, we call this process "neurological repatterning," which is really just a fancy phrase for changing beliefs.

Effectively, this process works to rewire your mindset and its associated beliefs so the next time you have a sexual encounter, instead of manning down you'll be manning up!

Essentially these newly empowered beliefs function as a "pattern interrupt" - they interrupt the negative cycle and create positive results. Remember, as you think, so shall you become, and right now it's time to become something much more than you've ever imagined by rewiring your brain with a new belief about sex.

To do this we are going to create a "New Belief Declaration" using a Circle of Results Model. First, both you and your partner will need to write down what your old belief about sex was using a Circle of Results Model. Here are some examples:

Old Belief Example - Men

Belief: I used to believe that every time I got naked with my woman my soldier would hibernate and lead to loads of embarrassment.

Thought: I thought... what is going on, why can't I get a hard on, what is wrong with me?

Emotion: I felt embarrassed, scared that I might be left alone.

Action: I bought some blue pills and when I got sick from taking them I gave in to the couch, binging on Netflix, ice cream and beer.

Result: My partner and I fought a lot and my relationship became a burden. I got depressed and put on extra weight.

Old Belief Example - Women

Belief: I used to believe that my man should be able to get an erection on his own regardless of his age. When he didn't get hard I thought he was just broken, that our sex life would never return and I lost faith in him and our relationship.

Thought: I thought... how did I end up with this broken man, did I pick the wrong guy, am I doing something wrong?

Emotion: I felt depressed, scared that I might be left alone.

Action: I told him he needed to fix his problem then drowned my own sorrows binging on Netflix, ice cream and wine.

Result: My partner and I fought a lot and my relationship became a burden. I got depressed and put on extra weight.

Time For Action - Write Down Your Old Belief

Now it's your turn to create a Circle of Results Model using your old belief. Go ahead and get out a pen and paper or write this in your electronic notes. Don't skip out here! This is where the real magic happens, where you begin to realize how your negative beliefs crush all hopes for a happy relationship, good sex, and youthful potency. Take action and start writing!

New Belief Declaration

Next, its time to take action and change this old belief with a newly empowered one. Let's take a look at a couple realistic examples:

New Belief Example - Men
Belief: I now believe my erection challenges are a natural part of aging and create an opportunity to strengthen my bond with my partner, have better sex and get even more love.

Thought: I think, wow, I get a new lease on life and I don't have to worry about getting an auto erection!

Emotion: I feel excited and empowered!

Action: I read this book with my partner, solve my core issues then try some of the team sex strategies.

Result: My partner and I have amazing sex, our relationship has never been stronger and it's translated into improving other areas like finances and overall health.

New Belief Example - Women

Belief: I now believe all men eventually have erection challenges which presents a great opportunity for couples to strengthen their bond with the magic of team sex.

Thought: I think... what a great opportunity to strengthen our bond and have amazing sex.

Emotion: I feel excited and hopeful!

Action: I read this book with my partner and tell him I'm 100% on board with team sex. We address the underlying causes of his ED and then try the team sex strategies.

Result: We have amazing sex and heal our relationship. Other areas of our life start to improve as well. I lost weight and I take better care of my health. I haven't felt this good in 20 years and I tell all my friends to go out and grab a copy of "Man Up!"

Time For Action – Write Down Your New Belief

Now go ahead and write down a new empowering belief about sex using a Circle of Results Model. Feel free to reference the example beliefs I created above then make sure you read the questions below, which will help you fine tune your beliefs.

Belief: What do you declare as your new belief?

_____

Thought: Describe the thoughts you'll have after you've embedded this new belief.

_____

Emotion: Describe how you will feel once this new belief is part of your permanent mindset.

_____

Action: What have you been unwilling to do in order to keep this problem? Describe the action you will take which will lead to a new habit.

_____

Result: How do you know for sure that your old belief is no longer a problem for you? Visualize your new outcome in detail – i.e., where will you be, who will be with you, any new habits created from the action, how will you feel?

Once you've written down your new belief in a Circle of Results Model its time to repeat it out loud at least 10 times.

Remember, "Repetition is the mother of all skill" so make sure you don't skip out on this challenge. If you don't repeat it, I can pretty much guarantee you won't remember it and your results most certainly will not change.

TIME FOR ACTION!

Now Repeat your own new belief to yourself out loud 10 times.

If you're at all doubtful how powerful your beliefs are in changing the results of your life you may want to consider one of the most comprehensive long-term studies on success ever conducted by Napoleon Hill which was featured in his book "Think and Grow Rich." As one of the top 10 best selling books of all time Hill unveils a remarkable discovery about the root cause of success and failure and its importance in history is significant.

After researching 500 of the most successful people in history over a 20 year period, Hill discovered that the cause of wealth and success had nothing to do with "money," "wealth," "finances," or "stocks." Instead, the most successful people attributed their success or the lack thereof to the psychological barriers (AKA beliefs). Hill's research culminated in one monumental statement as follows:

> *"Whatever The Mind Of Man Can Conceive And Believe, It Can Achieve."*

Yes, your mind is the most powerful tool in your arsenal and can not only determine how much money you make but how much soldier strength you have or don't have.

Again, what you think, you become and if you can change your beliefs and their associated thoughts you can completely change your destiny with increased wealth, improved health, stronger erections, and independent confidence nobody can ever take away from you. This brings us back to the most important question of this entire training:

Are You Taking Action?

Without action, your results will remain the same – man down! We can verify this by simply revisiting the Circle of Results Model. If you recall: beliefs lead to thoughts, thoughts lead to emotions, emotions lead to actions and actions lead to… results!

Ultimately, action is the bridge between your thoughts and results.   So let's say for example, you struggle with eating too much, working too much, not getting enough rest or not moving your body (all of which kill your testosterone and nitric oxide production) there's a really good chance you have a belief that prevents you from taking a new action.

Believe me, I know how difficult it is to do something different and change a habit that's been ingrained and conditioned over years if not decades. I used to get hungry about an hour or two before bed and to satisfy that little voice in the back of my head (give me more, give me more) I would munch on nuts, cookies or whatever happened to be in the kitchen at the time. But even though this created a ton of gut pain and stole precious sleep (man down) I continued doing it anyway.   Sound familiar?

Interestingly, the more I talked to people about breaking old habits, the more I realized how pervasive and challenging it was to actually change a belief long-term and create new results.

Fortunately, as we learned the masters of time mentioned earlier, in order to fix the root of any problem you must first address your beliefs.   This is the clear and simple reason why most diets and exercise programs fail – your beliefs!

Since changing your beliefs is so critical to solving the root of our problems, I set aside three years of my life and created perhaps the most effective and powerful brain rewiring system available called The Winner's Mindset.

Of course, no training is effective unless it gets long-term results, which is exactly what I got.   By simply pressing the play button and listening over and over (Remember repetition is the mother of all skill?) I've been able to change my belief about what food and sleep mean to me. And… I no longer eat late at night.

Instead, I've manned up, silenced that whinny kid and boosted my testosterone, nitric oxide and human growth hormone, which in turn has boosted my soldier strength to steel pipe and multiplied my income by 300%.

But I'm not the only one, this belief change system has helped hundreds of people rewire their brains for complete success in all areas of life including health, wealth and loving relationships. So if you have any challenges implementing these strategies, or you're at all curious, I highly recommend checking out some of those success stories and a free 90-minute video training at www.ChadScottCoaching.com. I guarantee you will thank me later.

Now hopefully you're even more hungry for success and open to our next Master Mantra from the sage and father of all medicine Hippocrates who famously declared:

"Let food by thy medicine and medicine be thy food."

This brings us to Chapter 9 "Mother Natures Master Miracles."

Chapter 9

Mother Nature's Master Miracles

Ok now that you've handled the most important element – your beliefs – and interrupted any negative thinking patterns, it's time to tap into Mother Nature's awesome power with some natural erection enhancers. Again, not to sound like a broken record, but if you just skip the root solutions like exercising, diet, team sex and most importantly your beliefs, I can guarantee one thing - your problem will keep returning like a nightmare that just won't end.

To make matters worse, if you haven't handled the root of your problem when you do take a supplement or even a PDE5 inhibitor, your body will be less responsive to their effects. Reason being, if you're toxic and/or overweight you're body will be working overtime trying to process and eliminate this toxicity.

A great analogy for such an obstruction is a nasty root that enters your kitchen pipes. Once it breaches a pipe, it begins to take over and clog the natural flow of activity. And once this happens, toxic sewage starts to back up and create all kinds of other problems, like smelly poo on your kitchen floor. (Not so fun!)

On the flip side, if you've handled the root and detoxified your body from overconsumption of refined sugars, alcohol and toxic chemicals, you'll most likely have shed any testosterone killing fat. When you get to this point and take a supplement or eat highly potent food, you'll feel the effects sharply magnified simply because that nasty root is no longer blocking the way for blood to flow through your pipes.

Time For A Reality Check!

Now before we jump in and get lost in the world of sexual stimulants, its time for a reality check! According to the National Institute for Aging, "quackery" is at an all-time high. Consumers are exposed to an overwhelming sea of advertising for dietary supplements and homeopathic products that promise instant relief of ED. Unfortunately, people blindly assume that some government entity, such as the FDA, has approved these products as safe and effective, which just isn't the case.

This widespread misconception has resulted in the spending of hundreds of millions of dollars for products whose efficacy has not been validated by clinical trials. In effect, many consumers are placing their trust in products promoted by manufacturers who do not invest the funds to carry out research to prove the safety and efficacy of these products.

So how do you find real, effective potent stimulants that aren't a waste of money?

The first rule of thumb is to stick to mother nature in her most pure state. As the old Motown song goes: "Ain't nothing like the real thing baby," and boosting your sexual potency is no different. So let's check out some of Mother Nature's Master Miracles.

Sunlight

Hundreds of studies have proven that natural sunlight triggers the production of vitamin D. But what's even more impressive is the fact that it also triggers the production of nitric oxide and serotonin.

For example, researchers at the University of Edinburgh found that when sunlight touches your skin, nitric oxide is instantly released into your bloodstream, which makes a lot of sense when you think about how good it feels to be in the sun. This study also found that sunlight exposure can significantly increase your life expectancy by cutting the risk of stroke.

Researchers concluded, "We suspect that the benefits to heart health of sunlight will outweigh the risk of skin cancer. The work we have done provides a mechanism that might account for this and also explains why dietary vitamin D supplements alone will not be able to compensate for lack of sunlight."

While a good vitamin D supplement is effective for many reasons, for instance, if you live in places where the sun just doesn't shine much, it's simply not a substitute for good old natural sunlight exposure.

For this reason, it's important to try and get around 15 minutes of sunlight exposure at least a few days per week. To do this you could sit with your shirt off and your back facing the sun or take a walk with your shirt off. Just make sure your face is protected with a hat or natural sunscreen.

Also, keep in mind, if you have naturally dark skin, you'll need around 20-30 minutes per day since your skin pigment doesn't absorb sunlight as quickly.

Mother Nature's Most Sexually Potent Foods

Once you get some free Nitric Oxide from the sun, it's time to step up to the plate, literally; as food, spices, and supplements from Mother Nature are some of your best options to get more of those two secret agents - nitric oxide (NO) and testosterone.

Nitric Oxide Foods (NO)

First off, food doesn't contain nitric oxide, instead, when you eat foods that contain natural nitrates, the bacteria in your tongue converts them into nitritines, and once you swallow the food, bacteria in your gut converts the nitritines into nitric oxide.

Now let's kick off this feast with some of the best vegetables and tubers (root vegetables) that boost nitric oxide.

- Leafy greens like spinach, arugula, kale, watercress, chervil

- Roots like beets pack a mean punch with more than 250 milligrams of nitrates per 100 grams (3.5 ounces).

- Runner up in this category with 100 to 250 milligrams per 100 grams is parsley, cabbage endive, fennel, leek, and celery.

Eat them RAW - According to a study by Oregon State University Extension, cooking these items can destroy their ability to increase your nitric oxide production, so if at all possible eat them raw in salads.

Beware Of Oxalates - As with all things in life, if you do something to the extreme and disregard balance you will have problems and eating nitrate rich vegetables is no different. Oxalates (or oxalic acid) are naturally occurring compounds found in vegetables.

Oxalates are antinutrients like those lectins we talked about earlier in wheat germ agglutinin which make you fat. Again, all plants have these lectins which function to protect against predators like insects, animals, and even humans.

Similarly, oxalates function to protect the plant and when you eat too many of these plants you can get kidney stones. But don't be alarmed, just make sure you eat a wide variety of these vegetables and consume spinach and beets in moderation as they contain 10x more oxalates that the majority of these nitric oxide boosting foods.

Add Nitric Oxide Vegetables To Most Meals!

These veges not only contain loads of nitric oxide but minerals, vitamins, and fiber, which are vital to your overall health and should be incorporated into every meal.

Omega-3 Fatty Acids

As one of the superstars of nitric oxide production and accompanying blood flow, omega-3 fatty acids are found mostly in fish and should also be a regular part of your diet. Interestingly, while most people have been brain washed into believing that fat makes you fat, according to Dr. Steven Gundry and Dr. Joseph Mercola, omega-3 fatty acids actually contribute to weight loss and reduce inflammation.

The challenge here is that our modern diet favors omega-6 fatty acids (processed vegetable oils, margarine, and trans fats) over healthy natural alternatives such as raw butter, olive oil, avocados, fish oil, cod liver oil and fatty fish like sardines and salmon. Don't fall into this trap! Make sure you eat high fat fish like sardines and salmon around 4-5 meals a week.

What Kind Of Fish Should I Eat?

When it comes to types of fish, make sure you choose species lower on the food chain, which will lower the amount of mercury intake, a highly toxic metal that deflates your soldier and defeats the whole purpose of this book.

For the most part, top of the food chain (high mercury containing fish) include fish like swordfish, shark, tuna and halibut. Make sure you shop with this in mind and stick to "wild caught" smaller fish with less mercury.

As for the land dwelling sources of Omega-3, focus on grass fed meat, raw butter, raw milk and ghee.

Buyer Beware!

Don't expect a whole lot if any Omega-3s from fish or cows that have been raised on corn and soy. Instead of Omega-3s, you'll be eating hormone disruptors and reactive lectins that throw your body way out of balance and kill all the work we've done so far. So again, stick to "wild caught" fish and "grass fed" meat if at all possible.

What If I'm Vegetarian Or Don't Eat Fish?

If you're vegetarian or just don't like fish there are other sources of Omega-3 fatty acids that come in vegan form but two of the most potent are walnuts (they don't look like testicles for no reason), hemp seeds and ground flaxseed.   All of these can be eaten as snacks (except late at night) or put on salads for a little extra boost of healthy fat and rich flavor.

Just keep in mind, it's extremely difficult to get enough Omega-3 fatty acids through a plant diet and you'll more than likely need to take a supplement. If this is you I highly recommend this trusty brand on Amazon - Nordic Naturals.

Best Sources Of Omega-3s:

Salmon, sardines, anchovies, mackerel, shrimp, lobster, grass fed meats, butter, ghee, walnuts, hemp seed and ground flax seed

Coenzyme Q10

Coenzyme Q10 (CoQ10) is a molecule found in the mitochondria of your cells, which produces energy. Just slightly important if you want to get out of bed in the morning, drive to work or use your brain. Joking aside, CoQ10 is critical for the health of your mitochondria and you'd be like burnt toast without it.

Unfortunately, as we age our natural production of this key molecule declines and low CoQ10 has been linked to male infertility, low testosterone, cardiovascular disease, fibromyalgia and Parkinson's disease.

Thankfully, supplementation and food sources with CoQ10 can increase your nitric oxide levels, relax your arteries and increase blood flow to your big guy. In fact, it's so important doctors like Dr. Joseph Mercola recommend it as one of the top 3 most important supplements to take daily.

First, let's check out some of the most potent CoQ10 foods, which should be incorporated into most of your meals.

Best Sources Of CoQ10:

Salmon, sardines, grass-fed meat, poultry, animal organs, egg yolks, Brazil nuts, and spinach.

Again, as you age, production of this valuable resource declines so if you're over 40 I highly recommend you grab a good CoQ10 supplement like Dr. Mercola's CoQ10 on Amazon

Quercetin

As one of the most researched flavonoids, Quercetin combined with other bioflavonoids like resveratrol, procyanidin, tannins, tea catechins, and genistein can pack a powerful punch and boost your nitric oxide levels.

Multiple studies have also proven that Quercetin improves your cardiovascular health by lowering systolic blood pressure, which is a sure sign of the presence of increased nitric oxide levels. Quercetin has also been found to directly increase nitric oxide output in corpus cavernosum ("body of the penis").[27]

While you can certainly buy supplements with Quercetin make sure you add some of the following foods to your main meals:

Best Sources Of Quercetin:

Onions, garlic, chives, kale, red leaf lettuce, asparagus, broccoli, cranberries

B Vitamins

B vitamins like B3 and B6 play a key role in sexual potency and can be found in a wide range of both food and supplements. Niacin (B3) is one of the 80 nutrients essential for human survival. To put it mildly, niacin plays a critical role in energy production, gene expression, and hormone synthesis - we simply can't live without it.

And yes... niacin increases nitric oxide synthase, and baseline NO levels with an added bonus of elevating your 'good' HDL cholesterol, while simultaneously lowering your 'bad' LDL cholesterol.[28] Sounds pretty darn good don't you think?

Again that should be consumed in most of your meals.

Best Sources Of B Vitamins:

Tuna, sardines, sweet potatoes and avocadoes

As you may have noticed, fish contains many of Mother Nature's most powerful penile potency elements. Accordingly, they should be on the menu several nights a week.

If for any reason you just can't muster the magic of fish, try piling on some spicy fat with cayenne and avocado, which will double up on your boner boosting power. Why?

Let's start with a fun fact: "Avocado" is derived from an Aztec word meaning "testicle." And yes they are good for your testicles or at least those baby soldiers that come out of them. Versatile and nourishing, avocados are loaded with vitamin E, which according to the National Institutes of Health is a key antioxidant that widens blood vessels, potentially lowering the risk for cardiovascular disease and may also reduce sperm DNA damage.

Avocados are also rich in vitamin B-6, which helps keep your nervous system in balance, potassium, which powers up your libido as well as monounsaturated oleic acid, which supports circulation and makes your heart healthy.

But that's not all! Avocados contain fat soluble vitamins A, D, E, and K, but also contain the fat helps you absorb them. So remember this one:

An Avocado A Day Keeps ED Away!

Zinc

As one of the most essential minerals, zinc is also key for sexual function because it helps your body produce testosterone as well as synthesize thyroid hormones necessary for energy production.

Some of the most potent forms of zinc include items we already covered so you may want to double down on these.

Best Sources Of Zinc:

Shellfish, red meat, nuts, raw dairy, and eggs

Raw Cacao

Cacao is the predominant ingredient in chocolate, which comes from cacao beans. When eaten in it's raw form, its is considered a superfood, which can give you a quick blast of nitric oxide and relax the inner lining of your arteries - good for blood flow to the big guy. The bonus here, especially in raw cacao, is that it contains loads of antioxidants and polyphenols, which protect you against the ravages of inflammation and old age.

If at all possible I recommend you purchase raw cacao, otherwise it will be processed with heat and destroy most of the antioxidants. You can buy raw cacao powder and put it in your smoothies or on yogurt. If you take this route I recommend a reputable brand like this one from Amazon.

If you're more inclined to much on straight chocolate bars for dessert or right before you have sex, which I highly recommend, try my personal favorite Raw Chocolate bars on Amazon.

Yes, you can eat regular chocolate that has been processed; just know that it will be less effective. And if at all possible make sure it contains over 70% cacao and does not contain soy lecithin (soy is a reactive lectin and hormone disruptor).

Coffee and Caffeine

While you may love your morning coffee or black tea, it may not love you back quite like you want it to. As you know by now, to get old stiffy back up to speed, you need more and nitric oxide, which dilates your blood vessels and lowers your blood pressure.

Sadly, the high caffeine content in coffee and black tea does the opposite. Instead of increasing blood flow it constricts it and raises your blood pressure. To top it off, caffeine is highly acidic and can create a breeding ground for candida and other energy sapping, Testosterone lowering bacteria and fungus.

And while coffee does contain antioxidants, which facilitate an increase of the enzyme nitric oxide synthase, which converts arginine into NO, the drawbacks mostly nullify these benefits. For this reason, you'll need to really lower your caffeine consumption and opt for decaf or green tea whenever possible.

Again, changing old habits isn't so easy. So not only do I recommend The Winners Mindset to change your beliefs about coffee and health, but I recommend trying some green teas like matcha or yerba mate, which can taste like coffee without the overload of caffeine. Here's a great option, which gives you 75 cups of tasty brew for $10 on Amazon.

Probiotics

Most health experts estimate that roughly 70% of you're your immune system is housed in your gut wall. And while probiotics have the power to create life and restore your natural gut bacteria, according to experts like Dr. Steven Gundry antibiotics indiscriminately carpet bomb your gut wall and wipe out both the bad and good bacteria.

So if you've been taking antibiotics for a long period of time or if you suffer from any gut issues, chances are you've wiped out a good chunk of your stomach soldiers and have an abundance of inflammation, which also means you are at high risk for heart disease. Unfortunately, as we mentioned earlier, heart disease is one of the main challenges of male potency and ED – man down!

This is really important for your health and understanding what is happening here can make a big difference in your soldier strength so listen up.

Essentially, your intestine's epithelial cells (cells that line the surfaces of your body) provide a physical barrier to pathogens and invaders and initiates an immune response when invaders attack. This is where probiotics come in huge.

Probiotics moderate the inflammatory response by repairing these epithelial barriers. They're like the infantry in your gut and support the production of anti-inflammatory short-chain fatty acids, and synthesize antimicrobial peptides. These "good bacteria" also affect molecules known as cytokines that can impact and reduce inflammation.

Without this burier of soldiers, the enemy would most likely overrun your defenses. Your gut and other body parts like joints and arteries will be on fire, literally. Unfortunately, all this inflammation can lead to ED and the most unsightly of scenes... Dead Dick!

To avoid this (assuming you've handled your root challenges) I recommend you eat fermented foods with every meal such as:

Best Sources Of Probiotics:

Yogurt (low or no sugar), fermented vegetables, fermented apple cider vinegar, fermented dairy, fermented sourdough bread (no preservatives) and kimchi

As amazing as these foods are for building soldier strength they will most likely not be enough to repair any previous gut damage, so in addition, I recommend a good probiotic supplement.

Buyers Beware!

There are literally thousands of probiotic supplements to choose from but most are ineffective, low quality, overpriced powder that dissolves without ever getting down to your small intestine.

If you don't have a proven source, which you know works, Dr. Mercola, one of the most trusted sources of health has developed one of the most potent probiotic supplements. Check it out here on Amazon.

Potent Spices From Mother Nature

There are several spices, which boost nitric oxide and increase blood flow but the two superpowers, which stand out and dominate this scene are Garlic and Capsaicin (Cayenne).

Garlic

We mentioned garlic in our Quercetin section, but it packs a remarkably powerful punch and can be used as a spice in your food so let's break down this tasty staple.

Garlic is chock full of nitrates, but also contains Quercetin, which as you know by now has also been linked to increased NO levels when consumed.

Several studies have also found that garlic is more effective at lowering blood pressure than most pharmaceutical drugs on the market. In one study, researcher Adam Moussa, gave his human subjects 2,000 mg of vitamin C along with 4 garlic tablets (6 mg of allicin and 13.2 mg of alliin) for 10 days.

At the end of the study, endolethial nitric oxide output increased by a whopping 200%, while on average patients systolic blood pressure dropped from 142 mm to 115 mm. And last but not least, Diastolic Blood pressure decreased on average from 92 mm to 77 mm. (Note: This beats most pharmaceutical drugs hands down)

One of the most important benefits of garlic supplementation is that it has been proven to kill off candida, which can sap your energy and send your soldier into hibernation. While it can obviously be incorporated into your meals, to really get garlic's boner boosting power you'll need to step up here and get a supplement like the one used in the example above. One of the most trusted brands in the garlic supplementation business which offers a Garlic and Vitamin C combo is Kyolic found here on Amazon.

Capsaicin / Cayenne

Capsaicin is the alkaloid that makes all chilies hot. It's literally the compound that creates a zap of heat in your mouth when you eat jalapeno pepper. But most importantly, it's also quite effective at increasing nitric oxide levels.

While you can eat chilies and add them to your food, keep in mind, there are toxic lectins in the skins and seeds of peppers, which is why I recommend you either buy them marinated with no seeds and skins or buy some cayenne pepper and sprinkle it on your food.

But why stop there? You can buy supplements that will magnify the power of cayenne like "Cool Cayenne" on Amazon, which adds ginger to prevent any gastric issues associated with too much of the fiery stuff. This high potency formula is really powerful and not only boosts nitric oxide and blood flow but will clean out toxins as well.

Remove The Obstructions

We've talked briefly about some problematic foods like whole grains which contain WGA, but in order for your body to regain its natural balance and actually use any of Mother Nature's potent foods and supplements it's absolutely crucial to eliminate things that block your production of Nitric Oxide and Testosterone and kill the blood flow to your big guy.

According to Dr. Steven Gundry, endocrine disruptors can block your body's natural healing process and lead to disease and dysfunction. To make sure you don't fall prey to some of these toxic foods make sure you eliminate the following from your diet:

- **Processed Meats, Poultry & Fish** – If at all possible, eat grass fed and wild caught fish without chemicals or preservatives.

- **Whole Grains** - Lectins like WGA and Gluten can cause weight gain and heart disease. Instead try sweet potatoes, white rice or millet in limited quantities

- **Artificial Sweeteners** – Several studies show that artificial sweeteners like Splenda, NutraSweet, Sweet 'N Low, Equal and Aspartame can lead to diabetes, atherosclerosis, IBS and addiction to sweets which makes you even fatter. Instead, try raw honey or stevia in limited quantities.

- **Give Fruit The Boot** - Too much fructose from fruit and fruit juice creates inflammation, weight gain and can lead to diabetes and heart disease! Instead, try berries or chocolate in limited quantities.

When it comes to food this is really just the tip of the iceberg when it comes to male potency killers and since it's such a detailed subject, again I highly recommend you read Dr. Steven Gundry's "The Plant Paradox," which has helped thousands of people lose weight and gain more youthful potency without having to give up tasty foods. Here's a link to that book on Amazon.

What About Vitamins?

Even if you've handled the root of your challenges and cleaned up your diet, sadly, the amount of vitamins and minerals in food will most likely be insufficient to grow and sustain your army of soldiers.

So What's Wrong With My Food?

A big part of the problem comes from years of poor farming practices, which according to a landmark study are "designed to improve traits (size, growth rate, pest resistance) other than nutrition."[29]

Sadly, today's agricultural practices (predominantly in the US) place a much greater emphasis on size over quality. (Can I get a big gulp? Or how about a King size snickers?)

Essentially, the soil in which most of our food is grown (particularly in the United States) is rarely enough to supply you with even the recommended daily allowances, which are low to begin with.

Since we know we need minerals like Zinc and Vitamins like B3 for boosting nitric oxide and testosterone, it's absolutely crucial to take a multivitamin, which includes these key vitamins and minerals.

Again, there are a multitude of options out there, but very few use pure whole food ingredients, which come from Mother Nature and actually work. So to make sure you don't get suckered into buying expensive urine pills, make sure you choose a "whole food multivitamin" that is not made of synthetic (unnatural) compounds.

Basically, if it doesn't say 100% whole food vitamin, then don't buy it; you'll just be wasting your money.

If you're short on recommendations, the most highly reputable brand, which I personally use, also happens to be a [best seller on Amazon](#) and again comes from Dr. Mercola.

L-Citrulline / L-Arginine

L-citrulline is an amino acid made by your body and contained in certain foods, which is converted by your body into another type of amino acid L-arginine.

If you're in the fitness world or read the trades you may have noticed the popularity of these amino acids - and for good reason. Several studies show they can significantly improve both resistance and endurance training.

For example, in one study, scientists from the University of Cordoba demonstrated how supplementation with 8 grams of L-citrulline before a chest workout increased the number of reps participants could do by 52 percent with an added bonus of significantly reducing postworkout muscle soreness.[30]

But What Is It That Provides The Boost Of Power?

Unsurprisingly, it's none other than that highly coveted secret agent of boner boosting power - nitric oxide. Yes, L-citrulline, which is converted to L-arginine produces significant quantities of nitric oxide and as you by now, nitric oxide increases blood flow to the big guy – man up! [31]

How To Get L-Citrulline

L-citrulline is most abundant in foods like meat and nuts. Quite ironic when you think about it - eat meat and nuts and your meat and nuts will thrive!

But that's not all! Several foods contain L-citrulline but I've narrowed the list to avoid sugary fruits like watermelon and legumes, which can lead to inflammation. If you are vegetarian and need to get your L-citrulline from legumes and beans I highly recommend you at least pressure cook or buy pressure cooked versions, which will remove reactive lectins that could potentially create leaky gut syndrome if not prepared correctly. And again, if you're curious about learning more about reactive lectins and why you should avoid them check out The Plant Paradox."

To get the most L-citrulline into your diet I've created a shortlist of foods that should be on your plate daily.

Meat   - preferably organic and grass-fed
Fish   - preferably wild caught low on the food chain
Nuts   - preferably skinless almonds and walnuts
Onion - preferably organic
Garlic - preferably organic

While you should be eating these foods daily, in order to recreate those studies and get enough nitric oxide to boost a steel pole you're most likely going to need to take a supplement. When you look online you'll find hundreds of choices but again, quality is really important here as fake products with fillers are the norm, not the exception.

How Much Should I Take?

The second thing you'll need to consider is the dosage. While I do recommend starting with the "recommended dosage" on the label, you'll need to experiment and see what your body can tolerate. If you've have handled your root problems of ED and do not have any risk of heart disease I recommend ramping up towards 8 -10 grams per day until you notice some boner boosting power.

There aren't a ton of long-term studies on supplementation so I would not take this every day. Instead, rely on your meat and nuts and supplement an hour or two before you know you'll be jumping in the sack.

While you can take this in pill or powder form I recommend trying "Doctors Best" powder form and adding it to water or a smoothie. Its virtually tasteless and odorless don't worry about what you take it with. Here's a link to that on Amazon Doctors Best L-Citrulline.

Chapter 10

Mother Nature's Turbo Chargers

There are literally thousands of male potency supplements on the market. But be forewarned, none of them will give you the power to raise a steel pipe on command like when you were 25. That said, there are some powerful plants that have been discovered, which have restored sexual potency to thousands of men and could be just what you need to top off your man up protocol.

In a nutshell, the supplements that I'm going to share will significantly improve your endolethial function, which allows for vascular relaxation, nitric oxide production and plays a large role in boosting blood flow, lowering blood pressure and boosting your big guy – naturally!

But... I need to issue another WARNING!

If you're experiencing testosterone deficiency and have yet to handle the root of your challenges, none of this will make much of a difference. Low T will decrease your nitric oxide production, plummet your libido and deflate your dong along with some other not so fun stuff like nasty arterial plaque and jacked up insulin.

Again, handle the root before you try any of these supplements. Be realistic here and don't look for miracles as these natural supplements take time to work and will function similar to foods and spices, which will boost your body's natural ability to produce an erection.

Red Korean Ginseng

Red Korean Ginseng, unlike a lot of other supplements, has several respected ED studies under its belt and could soon be one of your most trusted allies.

Best known as an adaptogen, Ginseng is an herb that supports your endocrine system to overcome stress while simultaneously giving you energy. What's remarkable about this energy boost is that is doesn't drop you off a cliff like caffeine from coffee does once it loses its power.

Several studies prove the efficacy of Ginseng including a significant discovery published in the Journal of Urology in 2002. In this double-blind, placebo-controlled study of 45 men with moderate to severe erectile dysfunction, researchers found improvement in erectile performance scores and sexual satisfaction after treating patients with three daily doses of 900 mg of Korean red ginseng for eight weeks.

Five years later, a similar study published in the Asian Journal of Andrology, resulted in all 60 male subjects reporting noticeable improvements in "rigidity, penetration and maintenance of erection." Most fascinating was the fact that these results only took 12 weeks using 1 gram of Ginseng per day.[32]

What Gives Ginseng Its Kick?

Panax ginseng (AKA Korean ginseng) contains active compounds called 'ginsenosides' which are structurally very similar to androgens, such as testosterone. Unsurprisingly, the rise in soldier strength from studies like the one just mentioned shows that Korean Ginseng increases testosterone and nitric oxide, improves circulation, promotes sleep quality, relaxes arteries, and boosts libido.

As you can imagine, with so many amazing benefits, ginseng is super popular, which also means that there's plenty of fake products on the market. So if you do decide to make a purchase just make sure you buy Korean Red Ginseng (Panax) not American or Siberian ginseng.

Most importantly, stay away from the fake stuff or check out my personal favorite on Amazon NutraChamps, which has yet to fail me.

Horny Goat Weed (HGW)

As one of the most popular ingredients in male potency formulas, Horny Goat Weed, like most other supplements, increases your nitric oxide production but also contains a flavonoid called icariin, which is known to mimic testosterone.

Numerous animal studies show how HGW makes rats "horny" and sexually active due to its active ingredient icariin, which naturally blocks PDE-5 enzyme similar to Viagra, Levitra, and Cialis. Realistically, while you won't get as much blood pumping through your magic wand as a pharmaceutical drug, a good dose of 100% pure organic HGW could do the job.

If you take this route just make sure to avoid products that are not 100% pure organic HGW or else you could end up with volcano butt and serious gas issues, especially if you have a sensitive stomach to begin with. If you'd like a recommendation here's a good reputable source on Amazon.

Muira Puama

Derived from the rainforests of Amazon, Muira Puama is similar to Horny Goat Weed and contains icariin as its active ingredient. In one noteworthy study, French sexologist Dr. Jaques Waynberg treated 262 men with Muira Puama who either had erectile dysfunction or libido issues. Two weeks into the treatment 61% of the men reported "dynamic improvements" and after a full month, 63% of the men reported that things were getting progressively better, with no side effects whatsoever.

The American Journal of Clinical Nutrition also reports that Muira Puama may have testosterone boosting effects in both men and women and could be a great choice, especially if you've had issues with HGW in the past or you know you have a sensitive stomach.

Again, if you take this round just make sure you don't buy a product with fillers and low grade Muira Puama compounds. Instead, check out this reputable brand of pure Muira Puama on Amazon.

Tribulus

Tribulus Terrestris is another super popular ingredient in male potency formulas and comes from a small leafy plant grown in parts of Europe, Asia, Africa, and the Middle East. Both the root and fruit of the plant have been used medicinally in Traditional Chinese Medicine and Indian Ayurveda medicine to boost libido and keep the urinary tract healthy. Does it work?

Researchers found that when men with reduced sex drives consumed 750 to 1,500 mg of Tribulus Terrestris daily for two months, their sexual desire increased by 79%. Women had a similar positive boost in libido with 67% of test subjects feeling increased sexual desire after they took supplements of 500 to 1,500 mg for 90 days.

Other studies have also reported that supplements containing the herb enhanced sexual desire, arousal, and satisfaction in women with low libido.

While this is good news (if you suffer from low libido or sexual desire), unfortunately, studies have found it does not reverse ED or increase testosterone to lift your soldier back to life. For these reasons, I recommend only using Tribulus as part of a broad-spectrum supplement, which we'll discuss shortly.

Maca

Maca is an Andean root, which resembles a radish or a turnip but tastes more like a potato. Like other starches, maca contains carbohydrates, protein, fats, and dietary fiber. It's also rich in plant sterols and is a good source of iron, magnesium, selenium, and calcium.

Georgetown University Medical Center professor Adriane Fugh-Berman, MD, says, "Some claims are over the top - compared to a placebo, maca only slightly enhanced sexual desire. The strongest evidence is that it may increase sperm count and improve fertility in certain men." Again, since this one on its own probably isn't going to give you a steel pipe erection on its own, I'm going to recommend it shortly as part of a broad spectrum potency formula.

Ashwagandha

Ashwagandha (Withania Somnifera) is an herb used in Ayurveda, the traditional medicine of India. Its root has a horsey smell and is said to confer the strength and virility of a horse. (In Sanskrit, ashva means "horse" and gandha means "smell")

Like Ginseng, Ashwagandha is an adaptogen, which helps your body adapt to stressors. Best known for its anti-anxiety properties, this herb can lower cortisol levels and may mitigate stress-induced insomnia, depression, and immunosuppression.

But Ashwagandha also has been shown to reduce low-density-lipoprotein cholesterol (LDL-C) and improve physical performance in both sedentary people and athletes.

While these are pretty impressive benefits, unfortunately, studies don't show a whole lot of steel pipe prowess. For example, one study published in AYU an international quarterly Journal of Ayurveda in 2011, less than 20% of participants using Ashwagandha had any change in ED symptoms. Researchers concluded, "Ashwagandha was not effective in the management of Psychogenic Erectile Dysfunction when compared with placebo."

Due to the lack of evidence of any steel pipe stiffness, again I'll recommend this one as part of a broad-spectrum supplement as it does have a lot of other quantifiable health benefits.

Pycnogenol & L-Arginine

Pycnogenol is a patented water extract from a flavonoid, which can be found in the bark of French maritime pine. L-Arginine is an amino acid that is used in the biosynthesis of proteins and helps your body produce nitric oxide.

In a study published in the Journal of Sex and Marital Therapy, a group of men suffering from erectile dysfunction were given L-Arginine and Pycnogenol. After one month of treatment with 1700 mg's of L-arginine per day, two of 40 male patients (5%) experienced a normal erection.

So L-Arginine may not be so hot on its own, but get this: when researchers treated patients with a combination of L-arginine and 40 mg of Pycnogenol twice per day for the second month, the number of men with restored sexual ability rose to 80%. Finally, after upping the dosage to 40 mg three times per day in the third month of treatment, 92.5% of the men experienced a normal erection.

Researchers concluded: "oral administration of L-arginine in combination with Pycnogenol causes a significant improvement in sexual function in men with ED without any side effects." These researchers believe that Pycogenol's additional benefits of lower blood pressure come from its ability to boost nitric oxide, which should come as no surprise.

Keep in mind, this stuff is really expensive and people get ripped off all the time by paying $100 plus for one bottle. Don't fall for this scam, here's a highly trusted brand NOW on Amazon that won't break the bank. As far as Pycnogenol in combination with L-Arginine, unfortunately, to my knowledge, there are none so I recommend a separate L-Arginine formula here.

Tongkat Ali / Longjack

Eurycoma Longifolia is a medicinal plant commonly referred to as Tongkat Ali (TA), Malaysian Ginseng or Longjack. Known as a traditional "anti-aging" remedy, TA has some of the most impressive studies of all which have shown the release of free testosterone, improved sex drive, reduced fatigue, and improved well-being.

In one of the more noteworthy studies, published in 2002 in the Andrologia Medical Journal, 200 mg of TA was given to 76 men suffering from late-onset hypogonadism (low testosterone) for one month. After treatment, 90.8% of the men showed normal testosterone levels with an average increase of just over 46%.

Another study published in the Journal of the International Society of Sports Nutrition not only showed a decrease in cortisol by 16% but an increase in testosterone levels by 37% in just four weeks.

Lastly, a study published in the British Journal of Sports Medicine gave 30 men between the ages of 31 and 52 100mg of TA for three weeks and found an increase in free testosterone in 73% of the men.

Ok, so Tongkat Ali clearly shows that it can boost the Big T, but remember it's also considered a libido booster and fat burner, which was demonstrated in a 12-week study on 109 men between the ages of 30 and 55. Evidenced Based Complementary and Alternative Medicine published this study and found TA supplementation to increase libido, erection strength, semen volume and significant fat loss.

If you take TA (Longjack) just make sure you read the recommended dosage as too much of this stuff can have negative side effects like insomnia and restlessness.   Again, this supplement can be way overpriced so don't just buy anything because it says its good. Here's a highly reputable brand of pure Longjack (Tongkat Ali) on Amazon.

Which Ones Should I Take?

At this point, you may be a little overwhelmed and I don't blame you; there's a ton of options out there! But don't worry; now that we've shed some scientific sunshine on the realities behind these supplements, we can narrow down the field and begin experimenting.

Below I've listed the 5 Rock Stars of pole boosting power, which stand above the rest and shown real proof of efficacy.

Top 5 Rock Stars of Pole Boosting Power

1) Tongkat Ali / Longjack
2) Red Korean Ginseng
3) Pycnogenol & L-Arginine
4) Muira Puama
5) Horny Goat Weed

Broad Spectrum Supplements

While you may want to buy a supplement that has all of these rock star pole boosters, I recommend not jumping the gun (pun intended) and blowing your wad of cash.   Just look at some of the reviews on Amazon for most of these products. Except for the fake reviews, most of them are horrible and show how much misguided information and advertising there is out there.

Why do most of these fail and have so many bad reviews?

Typically when broad spectrum supplements do not work it can be attributed to four main reasons as follows:

1) **It all comes back to the root.** A lot of these guys are looking for a pill to change their lives and simply aren't willing to do the work to weed out the root cause of erection dysfunction. Make sure you don't fall into this trap; handle the root cause first!

2) **The supplements are not from pure sources.** Impurities and additives can render these compounds useless or make your stomach do backflips with indigestion.

3) **You aren't taking the right dosage.** Too little won't do anything and too much could again make you sick.

4) **Your body may reject one of the elements in the formula.** Remember those lectins? Not all plants were meant to be eaten.

Based on the above studies, loads of testimonials and my personal experimentation here's my bottom line recommendation:

"Experiment With What Works For Your Own Body!"

Start Here First

We're all different, so make sure you don't just jump on the bandwagon and waste your money because someone else says it works. To take all of the guesswork out of what really works (especially if you have a sensitive stomach), start with one of the top 5 rock stars in its purest form and add it to smoothies or drink it with water. Just make sure you take it regularly at the manufacturers' recommended dosage for 2-3 months before you decide whether or not it's working.   Below are links to the purest forms of the top 5 rock stars:

1) Tongkat Ali / Longjack
2) Red Korean Ginseng
3) Pycnogenol & L-Arginine

4) Muira Puama
5) Horny Goat Weed

Second Option

The second option here is to try a much more natural broad-spectrum supplement which has a better chance at being effective since the ingredients are pure and the brand is more trusted. I recommend Nature Wise who sells a combo of Ashwagandha, Maca, Ginseng, Shilajit and Muira Puama. Here's a link to that product on Amazon.

Third Option

If you know your stomach is like cast iron and you digest stuff like a Billy goat then you may want to try one of these broad spectrum supplements, which contain most of the top 5 rock stars and has some of the best reviews on Amazon. Here's a great choice with Horny Goat Weed: Horny Goat Weed for Men & Women with L Arginine, Muira Puama, Maca Root, Tribulus
    Or try this one without Horny Goat Weed: Maca, Ginseng, Sarsaparilla, Muira Puama & Tongkat Ali

Cannabis

While cannabis continues to show promise for medicinal use, its progression into mainstream society has brought with it a mounting pile of studies, which testify to both its inherent benefits and drawbacks.[33]

First... The Good News!

A study published in the Journal of Sex Medicine analyzed 28,176 women and 22,943 men nationwide who were surveyed by the Center for Disease Control (CDC) via a questionnaire and concluded:

"Marijuana use is independently associated with increased sexual frequency and does not appear to impair sexual function." In fact, daily users across all demographic groups reported having 20% more sex than those who have never used cannabis.

The study further surveyed 289 adult women, and found that 65% claimed cannabis enhanced their sexual experience, 23% said it did not matter one way or the other, 9% had no significant feedback and 3% said it sabotaged their sexual experience.

Lead researcher Dr. Grover believes the enhanced sexual experience may be due to the "short-term anxiolytic (anxiety reduction) of cannabis." In other words, since anxiety and stress are usually linked to low libido in both men and women, at least in the short-term, cannabis can have the effect of reducing anxiety and enhancing sex.

The Bad News?

Unfortunately, according to studies, long-term use can increase anxiety, which may explain the lack of libido in habitual users.[34]

But let's not throw the baby out with the bathwater. If you rarely use cannabis and need a short-term boost from Mother Nature this could be just the right amount of magic to lift your wand up and solute her majesty.

But the potential benefits get even more interesting as scientists have proven that cannabinoids have an observable effect on the cardiovascular system, including raising resting heart rate, dilating blood vessels, and making the heart pump harder. As you know by now your dong needs more blood flow in order to get stiff, so this is good news, right?

The Pot Paradox

The paradox here is that cannabis can increase blood flow to your big guy but ongoing use can backfire especially if you have heart disease or are at risk of heart disease.[35]

According to Harvard Health Publications, "research suggests that the risk of heart attack is several times higher in the hour after smoking marijuana than it would be normally. While this does not pose a significant threat to people who have minimal cardiovascular risk, it should be a red flag for anyone with a history of heart disease."[36]

But again, there's no need to throw the baby out with the bathwater. If you've handled any potential challenges of cardiovascular disease, and you're not a habitual cannabis user, this could be a potential short-term solution to get your soldier back on duty.

Lastly, while some small studies have suggested that recreational marijuana use may lead to ED, authors of a 2018 meta-analysis concluded that there is not enough evidence to confirm a link.[37]

If this sounds like something that might work for you, you'll need to discuss it with your partner as part of your "Team Sex" talk. And if you don't have much prior experience with cannabis remember this one:

Start Low And Go Slow!

According to Michelle Ross, founder of IMPACT Network, a nonprofit organization that uses empirical medical research to find new cannabis-related treatments for patients, most people "just blast their system with cannabis or high amounts of THC, and that is not always the best approach for whatever condition they have."

Ross generally recommends that first time microdosers start off at 2.5 milligrams, maintain that level for approximately three days, and increase if necessary.

So start slow and if you live in a state that has legalized cannabis for recreational use make sure you ask the clerk for this specific dosage either in an edible or smokable form.

Chapter 11

The Biggest Bone Breaker Of All

Alas, we've come to the end of this book. But in reality, your journey is just beginning. Once you have a good idea of where the root of your personal challenges lie, it's time to man up and do that one thing that expands your capacity more than anything else – Take Action.

While your tendency may be to take the shortcut and go straight for a pill popping solution, if you're experiencing testosterone deficiency none of this will make much of a difference.

Low T will decrease your nitric oxide production, take away the magic from your wand and plummet your libido. So again, I highly recommend taking action towards getting your T back up first with a course like "Fired Up" and a diet regime like "The Plant Paradox."

But even more importantly, if you've failed with workout or diet programs in the past, guaranteed the underlying roots of your challenge lie not in your hammer but in your head - in your belief systems.

As mentioned in Chapter 8, without the right mindset, sticking to a diet or workout program will never work long-term, so if you've struggled with these in the past, you'll need to handle this with some specific action towards mental mastery.

Man Down?

Sadly, for most guys, this will be the end of the journey towards any potential restoration of sexually potency and manning up. Why?

Because the biggest life crusher and boner breaker for all men is that they simply don't the action to get help.

But hey, I'm a man... I get it! We men want to be independent. We are conditioned our whole lives to believe that asking for help is a sign of weakness. But in reality, nothing could be further from the truth - nothing!

Asking For Help Is A Sign Of True Strength, Not Weakness

Without seeking help your chances of becoming stronger, smarter, wiser or wealthier will remain just a dream. And let's not forget the biggest regret at the end of life:

Are You Just Doing What Others Expected Of You?

In order to flip this switch, live without regrets and experience a really exciting life, you'll need to, learn, grow, expand your capacity and see what you're really made of. This means taking action!

Without action and learning from others, the master goal of increasing your capacity is simply impossible.

So just know... if you have any challenges implementing the tools and strategies outlined in this book or would like more help, just know this:

I Got Your Back!

My goal in life is to help as many people as possible maximize their potential and as Jim Morrison from the Doors so famously said:

"Break On Through To The Other Side"

So if you're at all curious or want to learn what the other side feels like, the side where action is easy, energy is abundant, blood flows freely and wealth is multiplied, then I'd like to invite you to check out one of the most comprehensive mindset trainings ever created called: "The Winner's Mindset."

By simply pressing the play button, this training allows you to embed the mindsets of over 175 of the most successful people in history as your own. This includes masters from sports, business, arts, science, politics and philosophy like:

Richard Branson, Tony Robbins, Warren Buffet, Steve Jobs, Roger Federer, Wayne Gretzky, Lou Holtz, Marianne Williamson, Gandhi, Franklin Roosevelt, Rumi, Bob Marley, Leonardo da Vinci,

Albert Einstein, Thomas Edison, Stephen Hawking, Socrates, Buddha, Camus and over 150 others.

With the Winner's Mindset, nothing can hold you back from taking action. And once you take action, not only will your soldier stand tall and reclaim your manhood, but you'll take action on doing the things you love most instead of doing what others expect of you.

This is where the real magic of life happens, where your greatest dreams become a reality. This training constitutes my life's work and took me over 10 years to complete and I'd like to offer you a free 90-minute video training.

If this sounds interesting just head over to my website and check out the Winner's Mindset at www.ChadScottCoaching.com

Action + Persistence = Success!

Regardless of whether you join me in a future training, make sure you take action, be persistent and never give up. If you simply keep taking the action outlined in this book or any of my trainings you will get new favorable results. That's my guarantee!

The World Needs Your Help!

Lastly, before we part, if you've gotten anything helpful or enlightening from this book I'm going to assume you are to some degree grateful and would like to pass on your newfound knowledge. Or if you have feedback to improve this much needed guide, I'd imagine you'd like to share that with me.

As I mentioned at the beginning, ED has become a worldwide plague of mass proportions, which has stolen the manhood hundreds of millions of men. So I'd like to pose a very important question and opportunity to you as follows:

If you could help another guy avoid the pain of ED and the incredible embarrassment, rejection and powerlessness it creates, would you do it? What if it only took 60 seconds?

How so, you say?

Quite simply, by taking 60 seconds to leave a review, Amazon will take note and suggest this book to more men looking for solutions. And if you have feedback that can improve Man Up and help more guys you can share that as well.

Activate Your Super Hero Power

To be absolutely clear, my primary goal is way beyond just selling more books. The real payoff for me is to help as many men as possible rise up above the shame, embarrassment and powerlessness of impotence. Nothing feels better than when I get an email from a reader who tells me they've used this guide to get rid of ED and bring more love into their lives.

This is what gets me out of bed in the morning and what has been scientifically proven to keep both of us out of the graveyard of broken dreams (Remember that #1 regret at the end of life).

If you've read my book "Get High On Confidence" you may recall the 3rd and most powerful level of confidence, "Superhero Confidence," which of course, is all about being a force for good. So by helping someone else, you'll not only be acting as a force for good but you'll gain a little bit of that Superhero confidence as well!

Plus, we cannot underestimate the power of a simple 60-second review as demonstrated in books like "The Power Of Now" and "The 5 Love Languages," which have helped millions of people because of reviews. Your support of Man Up can do the same.

How To Leave A Review

1) Visit www.ChadScottCoaching.com/manup and you'll be automatically redirected to the book, then scroll down until you see "Write a customer review." Make sure you're logged in or it won't be a verified review.

    Or

2) Go to www.Amazon.com and search for "Man Up by Chad Scott" click on the book, then scroll down until you see "Write a customer review." Make sure you're logged in or it won't be a verified review.

Please share a quick sentence or two about what you learned along with any suggestions for future improvement so we can inspire more men to Man Up, live a life free of regrets and beat this plague. I look forward to your feedback and hopefully seeing you in a future training.

To your success, Chad Scott

Copyright © 2019 Chad Scott Nellis
All rights reserved. No part of this publication may be reproduced or transmitted in any form or by any means, electronic, or mechanical, including photocopying, recording, or by any information storage and retrieval system.

References

[1] Sexual dysfunction in the United States: prevalence and predictors. JAMA 1999 Apr 7;281(13):1174. Laumann EO, Paik A, Rosen RC

[2] The likely worldwide increase in erectile dysfunction between 1995 and 2025 and some possible policy consequences. BJU int. 1999 Jul;84(1):50-6 Ayta IA, McKinlay JB, Krane RJ

[3] 3 Courtenay WH. Behavioural factors associated with disease: injury and death among men: evidence and implications for prevention. Journal of Men's Studies. 2000;9:81–142

[4] Francome C. Improving men's health. London: Middlesex University Press; 2000. p. 6.

[5] BMJ. 2001 Nov 3; 323(7320): 1058–1060. No man's land: men, illness, and the NHS by Ian Banks

[6] The Seven Principles for Making Marriage Work by John Gottman, PH.D., and Nan Silver pg.265

[7] Statista - Average daily TV viewing time per person in selected countries worldwide in 2016 (in minutes)

[8] Thayer JF, Hansen AL, Saus-Rose E, Johnsen BH, Heart Rate Variability, Prefrontal Neural Function, and Cognitive Performance The Neurovisceral Integration Perspective on Self-regulation, Adaptation and Health Ann Behav Med. 2009,37(2):141-153. Doi10.1007/sI2160-009-9101-z.

[9] Segerstrom SC, Nes L.S. Heart Rate Variability Reflects Self-Regulatory Strength, Effort, and Fatigue. Psychol Sci. 2007;18(3)275-281. Doi:10.1111/j.1467-9280.2007.01888.x; Taylor CB. Depression, heart rate related variables and cardiovascular disease. Int J psychophysiol. 2010;78(1);80-88. Doi:10.1016j.ijpsycho.2010.04.006

[10] Berns GS, McClure SM, Pagnoni G, Montague PR, Cohen JD. Predictability modulates human brain response to reward. J Neurosci. 2001.21(8).2793-2798. Doi:10.1523/jneurosci.4246-06.2007

[11] Steidle, C.P. et al. "Correlation of Improved Erectile Function and Rate of Successful Intercourse with Improved Emotional Well-Being Assessed with the Self-Esteem and Relationship Questionnaire in Men Treated with Sildenafil for Erectile Dysfunction Stratified by Age," Current Medical Research and Opinion (2006) 22:939.

[12] Viagra Falls: Older Men Aren't Very Into Erection Drugs Michael Castleman Psychology Today Mar 01, 2016

[13] Banner, L.L. and R.U. Anderson. "Integrated Sildenafil and Cognitive-Behavior Sex Therapy for Psychgenic Erectile Dysfunction: A Pilot Study," *Journal of Sexual Medicine* (2007) 4(4, Pt 2):1117.

[14] Annals of Internal Medicine, August 2003. News Release, American College of Physicians.

[15] Pathophysiology of Hypertensive Renal Damage Implications for Therapy Anil K. Bidani and Karen A. Griffin published Nov 2004

[16] Meulener, M. Current Biology, Sept. 6, 2005; vol 15: pp 1572-1577. News release, Cell Press.

[17] Prevalence of sexual dysfunction in male subjects with alcohol dependence Bijil Simon Arackal and Vivek Benefal Indian J Psychiatry. 2007 Apr-Jun; 49(2): 109–112.doi: 10.4103/0019-5545.33257

[18] Cigarette Smoking and Erectile Dysfunction: Focus on NO Bioavailability and ROS Generation J Sex Med. Rita C. Tostes, PhD,* Fernando S. Carneiro, MSc,*† Anthony J. Lee, PhD,‡ Fernanda R.C. Giachini, MSc,*†Romulo Leite, PhD,† Yoichi Osawa, PhD,‡ and R. Clinton Webb, PhD‡ 2008 Mar 4. doi: 10.1111/j.1743-6109.2008.00804.x

[19] Experimental Biology 2018. "Even a single mindfulness meditation session can reduce anxiety: People with anxiety show reduced stress on the arteries after 1-hour introductory session." ScienceDaily. ScienceDaily, 23 April 2018.

[20] Harman SM, Metter EJ, Tobin JD, et al. Longitudinal effects of aging on serum total and free testosterone levels in healthy men. Baltimore Longitudinal Study of Aging. J Clin Endocrinol Metab. 2001;86:724–31

[21] J Physiol. 2013 Feb 1; 591(Pt 3): 641–656. Published online 2012 Sep 3. doi: 10.1113/jphysiol.2012.239566 Sprint interval and endurance training are equally effective in increasing muscle microvascular density and eNOS content in sedentary males Matthew Cocks,1 Christopher S Shaw,1 Sam O Shepherd,1 James P Fisher,1 Aaron M Ranasinghe,2Thomas A Barker,2 Kevin D Tipton,3 and Anton J M Wagenmakers1

[22] "Yoga for anxiety: A systematic review of the research evidence. Br J Sports Med. 2005"

[23] PLoS One. 2007; 2(5): e465. Published online 2007 May 23. doi: 10.1371/journal.pone.0000465 Resistance Exercise Reverses Aging in Human Skeletal Muscle Simon Melov,#1, * Mark A. Tarnopolsky,#2, * Kenneth Beckman, 3 Krysta Felkey, 1 and Alan Hubbard 1

[24] The Seven Principles for Making Marriage Work by John Gottman, PH.D., and Nan Silver pg.100 and 265

[25] Effects of acutely displaced sleep on testosterone. Axelsson J, Ingre M, Akerstedt T, Holmbäck U J Clin Endocrinol Metab. 2005 Aug; 90(8):4530-5.

[26] EMBO Rep. 2006 Apr; 7(4): 358–361.doi: 10.1038/sj.embor.7400671 Science and Society Analysis Mind–body research moves towards the mainstream, Vicki Brower

[27] Protective effect of resveratrol and quercetin on in vitro-induced diabetic mouse corpus cavernosum Charlotte Boydens, Bart Pauwels, Laura Vanden Daele, and Johan Van de Voorde

[28] Am Heart J. 2002 Jul;144(1):165-72. A novel mechanism for the beneficial vascular effects of high-density lipoprotein cholesterol: enhanced vasorelaxation and increased endothelial nitric oxide synthase expression. Kuvin JT, Rämet ME, Patel AR, Pandian NG, Mendelsohn ME, Karas RH.

[29] University of Texas (UT) at Austin's Department of Chemistry and Biochemistry was published in December 2004 in the Journal of the American College of Nutrition

[30] Perez-Guisado J, Jakeman PM. Citrulline Malate Enhances Athletic Anaerobic Performance and Relieves Muscle Soreness. J Strength Cond Res. 2010;24(5);1215:1222. Doi:10.1519/JSC.0b0I3e3181cb28el).

[31] Bescos R Surenda A. Tur JA, Pons A. The Effect of Nitric-Oxide-Related Supplements on Human Performance. Sport Med. 2012:42(2):99-117. Doi:10.2165/11596860-00000000-00000; Orozco-Gutiérrez JJ, Castillo-Martinez L. Orea-Tejeda A, et al. Effect of L-arginine or L-citrulline oral supplementation on blood pressure and right ventricular functions in heart failure patients with preserved erection fraction. Cardiol J. 2010;17(6):612-618; Cormio L, De Siati M, Lorusso F, et al. Oral L-Citrulline Supplementation Improved Erection Hardness in Men With Mild Erectile Dysfunction. Urology. 20111;77(1):119-112. Doi:10.1016fj.urology.2010.08.028.

[32] Spermatogenesis. 2013 Jul 1; 3(3): e26391. Published online 2013 Sep 13. doi: 10.4161/spmg.26391 Ginseng and male reproductive function Kar Wah Leung and Alice ST Wong*

[33] Association Between Marijuana Use and Sexual Frequency in the United States: A Population-Based Study Andrew J. Sun, MD1 Michael L. Eisenberg, MD

[34] Association Between Marijuana Use and Sexual Frequency in the United States: A Population-Based Study Andrew J. Sun, MD,[1] Michael L. Eisenberg, MD

[35] J Clin Pharmacol. 2002 Nov;42(S1):58S-63S. Cardiovascular system effects of marijuana. Jones RT

[36] Marijuana and heart health: What you need to know Published: August, 2017 Updated: June 24, 2019 Harvard Health Publication / Harvard Medical School

[37] J Sex Med. 2018 Apr,15(4):458-475. doi: 10.1016/j.jsxm.2018.02.008. Epub 2018 Mar 6. Health-Related Lifestyle Factors and Sexual Dysfunction: A Meta-Analysis of Population-Based Research. Allen MS Walter EE

Printed in Great
Britain
by Amazon